EVIDENCE-BASED

MANAGEMENT

IN HEALTHCARE

EVIDENCE-BASED
MANAGEMENT
IN HEALTHCARE

ANTHONY R. KOVNER, DAVID J. FINE,

RICHARD D'AQUILA

AUPHA

13   12   11   10   09   5   4   3   2   1

Library of Congress Cataloging-in-Publication Data

Evidence-based management in healthcare / [edited by] Anthony R. Kovner, David J. Fine, Richard D'Aquila.   p. ; cm.
  Includes bibliographical references and index.
  ISBN 978-1-56793-306-2
1. Health services administration--Decision making. 2. Evidence-based medicine. I. Kovner, Anthony R. II. Fine, David J. III. D'Aquila, Richard.
  [DNLM: 1. Health Services Administration. 2. Decision Making. 3. Health Policy. W 84.1 E933 2009]
  RA971.E983 2009   362.1068--dc22

                                                                    2008038716

The paper used in this publication meets the minimum requirements of American National Standard for Information Sciences—Permanence of Paper for Printed Library Materials, ANSI Z39.48-1984. ∞™

Project manager: Eduard Avis; Acquisitions editors: Janet Davis and Eileen Lynch; Book and cover designer: Scott R. Miller

Health Administration Press
A division of the Foundation
  of the American College of
  Healthcare Executives
One North Franklin Street
Suite 1700
Chicago, IL 60606
(312) 424-2800

Association of University Programs
  in Health Administration
2000 14th Street North
Suite 780
Arlington, VA 22201
(703) 894-0940

To Jack Karp, an evidence-based manager and a faithful friend.
–Anthony R. Kovner

❖

To Susan Marie Gory, whose husband I have had the good fortune to be.
–David J. Fine

❖

To my wife, Kathy, and my family—without their support for my career this would not be possible.
–Richard D'Aquila

BRIEF CONTENTS

III Case Studies of Management Interventions Using an Evidence-Based Management Approach

IV Lessons Learned, and Where Do We Go from Here?

V Supplementary Materials

DETAILED CONTENTS

FOREWORD: THE IMPORTANCE OF ADOPTING EVIDENCE-BASED MANAGEMENT IN HEALTHCARE

For healthcare to be safe, effective, efficient, and reliable, people involved in the healthcare system need to get a lot of things right—not just the individual clinical decisions about prevention and care for each patient, but also the management and policy decisions about how to organize, manage, and pay for that care. As a nation, we have come to embrace the truth that getting the clinical decisions right requires wide-scale application of the principles of evidence-based medicine. We are only now, late in the game, recognizing that systematic use of evidence also could improve the big decisions affecting care throughout a hospital, health plan, physician practice, nursing home, or community. In fact, successful implementation of evidence-based medicine requires the support of evidence-based management. *Healthcare can be only as good as the system that provides it*, and therefore true improvement will require us to embrace evidence-based management.

This book, bringing together the thoughts of health services researchers and healthcare managers—a significant feat in itself—provides important conceptual thinking and illustrative case studies to help move us in this direction.

Widespread application of evidence-based management will not be easy or quick. The history of evidence-based medicine is long and tortuous, and achieving evidence-based management is likely to be even harder. Indeed, managers may find much of the conceptual foundation for evaluating clinical interventions irrelevant. Biology does not exhibit local variation the way physician practices or hospital or health plan administrations do, and the assessment of strategies and programs can rarely be standardized. Attempting to reproduce the successes of one setting in other locations will bring new insights and challenges, since the variability in organizational characteristics is likely to influence the outcome. In addition, the methods and tools likely to yield fruitful results are fairly nascent.

Forward progress will require innovative approaches and their application in a context of considerable urgency, as the challenge to deliver care that is safe, high quality, and efficient continues. As several of the chapters point out, progress will depend on attitude changes and transformed educational strategies among healthcare leaders and managers.

We recognize the imperative of achieving a far more impressive return on the substantial expenditures allocated to healthcare. At the Agency for Healthcare Research and Quality, we have spent several years obtaining systematic input from users (and nonusers) of management evidence and calibrating our research initiatives to attempt to meet the needs of health system leaders and managers. Enthusiasm for celebrating the chapters here should be tempered by a clear-eyed appreciation of the challenges inherent in embedding evidence in all aspects of healthcare delivery.

Description is not the same as problem solving. Descriptions and trend data are extraordinarily useful as ways to identify an issue, and even as a "call to arms." For example, the impact of the Institute of Medicine's identification of almost 100,000 deaths per year from medical errors cannot be overstated. To act on evidence, however, managers need information at a much more granular and actionable level—what kind of system change, with what kind of implementation strategy, is likely to reduce which kind of error? Actionability will be a key requirement in future research.

Actionability or utility must be informed by managers' needs for information and beliefs regarding that information. Researchers might believe they are in the best position to make an educated and neutral definition of what constitutes "good evidence," but those who are making management decisions often have good reasons for holding a contrary view. For example, research may show what works *most* of the time, but decision makers need to know what is likely to work in their particular circumstances. In this situation, asking for advice from colleagues in similar institutions may be more rational than consulting cross-sectional data analyses.

The imperative to change healthcare delivery dramatically has been articulated in numerous reports from authoritative bodies. Inquiries intended to illuminate how managers can transform a "broken" system are a leading frontier of healthcare research. Collaborative work between researchers and managers—as in this book—is likely to be particularly effective in achieving evidence-based management. Of particular note, the urgency perceived by managers to do "something" now should not be an excuse to overlook the impact of system changes. Understanding both the interventions that worked and those that failed to achieve their promise (and *why*) will be essential to improving healthcare delivery on a scale that is desperately needed. In addition, as this text shows, encouraging healthcare leaders to use evidence in their decision making is likely to require changing the educational and accrediting systems in which they operate.

This book makes an important contribution to the field by focusing on how managers can and do use the evidence we have. An appropriate next step for all invested in healthcare is to seek ways to broaden such practices and expand the knowledge base, so that evidence-based management becomes the rule rather than the exception. We look forward to working with all stakeholders to help make that happen.

Irene Fraser, PhD
Director, Center for Delivery,
Organization and Markets,
Agency for Healthcare Research and Quality

Carolyn M. Clancy, MD
Director, Agency for Healthcare
Research and Quality

December 2007

ACKNOWLEDGMENTS

Without the significant contributions of many talented and pioneering individuals who have taken on the challenges of making important decisions in healthcare delivery based on the process and techniques of evidence-based management (EB management), this book would not exist.

At the top of the list of people whose efforts we wish to acknowledge are the case writers: Philip DiSalvio; Ann Scheck McAlearney; K. Joanne McGlown, Stephen J. O'Connor, and Richard M. Shewchuk; Patricia Gail Bray; Arthur Webb and Ellen Flaherty; Kyle L. Grazier; Kenneth R. White and J. Brian Cassel; Lawrence Prybil, William Murray, Timothy Cotter, and L. Edward Bryant, Jr.; Jancy Strauman; and Megin Wolfman.

We also are indebted to the authors of the other chapters in this book: Irene Fraser, Carolyn Clancy, Thomas G. Rundall, Peter F. Martelli, Rodney McCurdy, Ilana Graetz, Laura Arroyo, Esther B. Neuwirth, Pam Curtis, Julie Schmittdiel, Mark Gibson, John Hsu, and Sara Mody.

We would also like to recognize the contribution and special efforts of authors of chapters and cases in the Instructor's Guide. These include case writers Jeffrey Bockser, Kathleen Gallo, Leonard Friedman, Kelley Kaiser, and Cynthia Struke. Also included are authors of special chapters on the implications of EB management for education and for management research. These authors are David Fine, Emily Garrison, Elester Stewart, Anthony R. Kovner, and Richard D'Aquila (on education), and Stephen Shortell, Thomas Rundall, Douglas Conrad, and Anthony R. Kovner (on research).

We have special appreciation for the hard work of our very capable assistants: Megin Wolfman, Emily Garrison, and Sara Mody. They are an unusual trio of tomorrow's stars and contributed greatly to whatever success this book achieves.

We would be remiss in our expressions of appreciation if we did not acknowledge the inspiration provided by the late Jeptha Dalston. Like us, Jep believed that those who teach and do research and those who practice management have a great deal to learn from each other. Tom Rundall deserves special thanks for the intellectual underpinnings for this work and for his consistent patience and courtesy.

We were fortunate to have the services and advice of a remarkable editor, Victoria Weisfeld, whose invisible footprints lie all over this text. And we thank Audrey Kaufman and three anonymous reviewers for their extensive and focused comments that helped shape this book.

Our funders were invaluable in helping us improve the quality of our work. They include Jack Karp and another donor who prefers to remain anonymous.

Tony Kovner would like to thank his colleagues at NYU/Wagner, particularly Ellen Schall, Dennis Smith, John Billings, and Steve Finkler and many of his outstanding students.

Finally, although too often it "goes without saying," we thank our spouses for putting up with us: Kathleen D'Aquila, Susan Gory Fine, and Christine Tassone Kovner.

April 2008

INTRODUCTION: ON THE PRACTICE OF EVIDENCE-BASED MANAGEMENT

Anthony R. Kovner, Richard D'Aquila, and David J. Fine

> *Evidence-based practice is a paradigm for making decisions that integrate the best available research evidence with decision maker expertise and client/customer preferences to guide practice toward more desirable results (Rousseau 2006).*

Our Intent

We wrote this book to share the experiences we and others have had in reflecting on and practicing evidence-based management (EB management). The book can serve as a text for a capstone course emphasizing EB management and as an invitation to healthcare organizations to practice EB management. We also hope to encourage healthcare organizations to fund EB management research initiatives. We assume that those who manage and those who teach management and do management research have a lot to learn from each other.

We have not written this book as an academic exercise. Nor have we merely presented practitioner war stories. The ten case studies in this book were written by managers and researchers involved in management interventions using some approximation of the evidence-based approach, sometimes retrospectively superimposing the EB management framework on already existing initiatives. We believe discussion and analysis of these cases will encourage those who study and practice healthcare management to obtain higher-quality evidence on management issues and to use it more effectively. The benefits of using an EB management approach—especially the longer-term benefits—often far outweigh the costs. You will read about some of these benefits in the case studies. Bad decisions, which can cost hundreds of thousands of dollars, may be avoided by spending the extra time and usually minimal financial resources on the EB management process.

A Scenario

Imagine the situation confronting the CEO of a 1,450-bed, 40-year-old urban hospital that is operating at full capacity and has a 10 percent market share in its region of 2 million people. The CEO must decide whether to recommend to the trustees that the main facility be rebuilt, and if so, whether to build satellite facilities and where they should be located. These decisions are complicated and costly, with many consequences, and different managers would approach them in different ways.

Alfred's approach: CEO Alfred hires three sets of consultants to bid on a planning project, reads several business books on strategic planning, and attends one or two professional meetings with sessions on this topic. Alfred discusses strategic planning with members of his board and the medical staff, management colleagues, CEOs of other hospitals, the president of the state hospital association, and major insurers. The information Alfred obtains from these sources does not always jibe, although all advisers agree that to stay competitive, Alfred has to rebuild his main facility at some time in the near future.

Barbara's approach: In the same situation, a second CEO, Barbara, considers acquiring a neighborhood community hospital that is operating at 60 percent capacity, losing substantial money, and providing uneven quality of care. Her strategy is to serve low-acuity hospital patients there, instead of at the main facility. State regulators are urging her to take over the community hospital. If the hospital goes under, this takeover will worsen healthcare access problems for its underserved neighborhood. The regulators have suggested financing the takeover with state payback to hospital bondholders, and then raising the county hospital's reimbursement rates by 30 percent to equal those of the main hospital.

Chuck's approach: A third CEO, Chuck, reviews management research and websites on strategic planning and mergers in hospitals and health systems, visits best-practicing health systems, and talks with consultants and managers. Chuck seeks evidence on the changing demographics of different actual and potential markets for his hospital and on the competitive strengths and weaknesses of key hospital competitors. He also seeks evidence on the amount of financing required under different merger/alliance options, ways this money can be raised, and the share amount that must be raised from the main hospital's operations.

All three CEOs use evidence to choose and implement managerial interventions. The use of one approach does not preclude the use of another. Two approaches, or parts of all three approaches, can be used together. The approaches vary in terms of costs and benefits. This book hypothesizes that carrying out a process of evidence-based decision making, which may include all or only some of the activities referred to above, will lead to more informed decision making and better organizational results.

All management decisions are based on evidence of varying quality. Too often in this fast-moving field, decision makers rely primarily on what has worked before or on a superficial analysis. We are not suggesting that there is valid and reliable evidence that can be inexpensively obtained for every planned managerial intervention. At times there may be significant costs to obtaining the necessary evidence, and these costs may not always be justified. The real and measurable costs of EB management must be weighed against potential significant benefits over the longer term that may be hard to quantify or to attribute to the specific EB management intervention.

Nevertheless, the process of EB management is often valuable in itself, as it can focus management thinking. For example, managers might be cautious about merging with hospitals across town if mergers between adjacent hospitals are shown to be more likely to succeed. Deeper analysis may (or may not) reveal that the successes occurred because of physicians' greater willingness to change hospital affiliations to a nearby facility and patients' greater willingness to travel there for specialty services. Research may also show which services and marketing strategies contribute to a successful merger regardless of location. Without that depth of understanding, the decision is essentially a coin toss.

The following evidence-based, step-wise process is the core of EB management: (1) framing the question; (2) acquiring research information; (3) assessing the validity, quality, applicability, and actionability of the evidence; (4) presenting the evidence to those who must act on it; (5) applying the evidence to the decision; and (6) evaluating results. These steps are often described in slightly different ways, covering the same activities, or, as noted, combined as appropriate. We are not rigidly prescriptive with respect to an EB management methodology, however, and believe that a systematic approach is essential, regardless of the steps used to apply it.

Our Approach to Case Studies

This book presents ten case studies examining management interventions. They were written by researchers who are experienced case writers and by managers who have lived through the experiences they describe. We encouraged the case writers to present the perspectives of stakeholders who argued for other alternatives and/or had differing perceptions as to the costs and benefits of the proposed management interventions. We also encouraged them to be brief regarding the success or failure of the interventions. We were primarily interested in how and why managers made decisions regarding planned interventions. In many instances, these fresh case studies have not yet fully played out.

Audiences

The primary audiences for this book are students of healthcare management, teachers, researchers, and healthcare managers. For example, one of us (Kovner) uses EB management as a primary pedagogical method for a capstone course, in which teams of three to five graduate students develop management interventions for a client organization. The book can also be used in tandem with standard texts in healthcare management, such as those written by Griffith and White (2007), Shortell and Kaluzny (2000), and Kovner and Neuhauser (2004).

Plan of the Book

This book comprises five parts:

Part I. Transformation to Evidence-Based Management

This part begins with research findings from Rundall and colleagues regarding the reasons why managers do not use EB management more widely in healthcare organizations. Hospitals and other healthcare organizations in the United States can be said to be operating in a time warp; some are operating as if it were 1950, or 1975, or 2000, or 2025. D'Aquila, Fine, and Kovner present their own experiences in moving toward practicing EB management in their disparate institutions. Respectively, these institutions are Yale-New Haven Hospital (New Haven, Connecticut), St. Luke's Episcopal Health System (Houston, Texas), and Montefiore Medical Center (Bronx, New York) and Lutheran Medical Center (Brooklyn, New York).

Rick D'Aquila describes the culture of Yale-New Haven Hospital, where he has led several important management initiatives as chief operating officer, including strategic planning, resource allocation, quality and safety surveillance, and development of performance management and operational dashboard systems. David Fine describes efforts over three years to transform the management culture at St. Luke's, where he is CEO. Tony Kovner then shares his experience with how management decisions are made at Montefiore Medical Center, where he has served for 16 years as a management consultant—primarily helping physicians perform management jobs more effectively—and at Lutheran Medical Center, where he has served as a member of the governing board, also for 16 years. Kovner focuses on the gap between EB management in theory and in practice.

Part II. Theories and Definitions of Evidence-Based Management

This section examines the way EB management is being defined and applied, specifically reviewing:

• Various theories and definitions of EB management, the types of questions to which EB management can be applied, and the valuable research of Hsu and colleagues (2006) regarding implementation;

- The use of evidence-based decision making by physicians and nurses that has resulted in patient-care guidelines and related decision-support materials; and
- The use of EB management in business organizations, including health-care organizations in Canada and the United Kingdom.

Kovner and Rundall group the types of management issues to which EB management can be applied into three areas: core business transactions, operational management, and strategic management. The types of questions it can answer range from: "What methods for paying physician claims achieve speed, convenience, and accuracy requirements?" to "How can nurse absenteeism be reduced?" to "How do hospital mergers affect administrative costs?"

This section also reports on recent research to identify and explore factors associated with knowledge transfer between researchers and managers of health systems (Kovner 2005). The research focused on managers of five health systems and four types of decisions: selecting the indicators for success of diabetes management programs; strengthening the relationship between budgeting procedures and strategic priorities; selecting the operational metrics in managerial dashboards; and adapting compensation systems for managers of physician performance.

Hsu and colleagues conducted four discussion groups with senior managers and policymakers from public and private healthcare organizations, from which they developed a set of tools to help decision makers obtain and assess information for use in making decisions about potential management interventions. The Management Toolbox that resulted, an excerpt of which is abstracted here, describes the six steps in the EB management process.

Sara Mody has written a reference for students on how to search for evidence in the literature, using "improving governance in nonprofit hospitals" as an example.

Part III. Case Studies of Management Interventions Using an Evidence-Based Management Approach

The case studies describe the use of the evidence-based approach in managerial inventions, undertaken on a variety of topics and in a variety of institutional settings. The range of topics and diversity of institutions involved have been crafted to demonstrate the wide applicability of the EB management approach to problem solving.

Part IV. Lessons Learned, and Where Do We Go from Here?

We draw conclusions from the lessons learned in our own attempts to encourage EB management. We address how incentives in these organizations can be aligned with EB management priorities and how culture that strongly supports evidence-based *medicine* can be leveraged to favor the implementation of evidence-based *management*, too. The authors discuss their plans to spread EB management utilization in their own organizations. (Figure 1 shows where organizations should focus their efforts.)

Part V. Appendix

Sara Mody has written an appendix on selected sources of information on the evidence-based approach and related topics.

Instructor Resources

Instructor resources for this book are available online. Materials include instructor's notes on statistics, financial analysis, and management; curricu-

FIGURE 1
Evidence-Based Decision Making: Where to Focus for Improvement

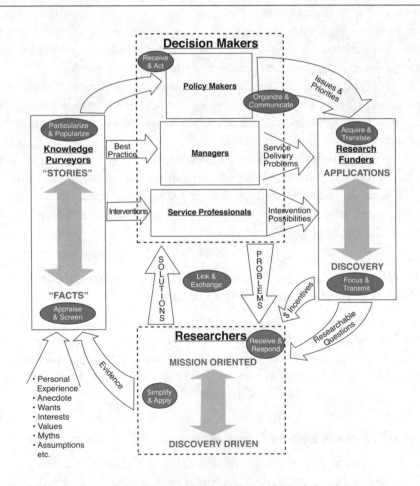

SOURCE: Reprinted with permission of the Canadian Health Services Research Foundation.

lum content; a syllabus for a capstone course; additional reading materials; and links to various websites. For instructions on how to access this information, e-mail hap1@ache.org.

References

Griffith, J., and K. White. 2007. *The Well-Managed Healthcare Organization*, 6th edition. Chicago: Health Administration Press.

Hsu, J., L. Arroyo, I. Graetz, E. Neuwirth, J. Schmittdiel, T. G. Rundall, and M. Gibson. 2006. *Methods for Developing Actionable Evidence for Consumers of Health Services Research (Match Study): A Report from Organizational Decision-Maker Discussion Groups & A Toolbox for Making Informed Decisions*, #290-00-0015. Rockville, MD: U.S. Agency for Healthcare Research and Quality.

Kovner, A. R. 2005. "Factors Associated with Use of Management Research by Health Systems." Unpublished report for the Center for Health Management Research. Seattle: University of Washington.

Kovner, A. R., and D. Neuhauser. 2004. *Health Services Management: Readings, Cases and Commentary*, 8th edition. Chicago: Health Administration Press.

Rousseau, D. M. 2006. "Is There Such a Thing as 'Evidence-Based Management'?" *Academy of Management Review* 31: 256–69.

Shortell, S., and A. Kaluzny. 2000. *Healthcare Management: Organizational Design and Behavior*, 4th edition. New York: Delmar Publishers, Inc.

THE TRANSFORMATION TO EVIDENCE-BASED MANAGEMENT

USING RESEARCH EVIDENCE WHEN MAKING DECISIONS: VIEWS OF HEALTH SERVICES MANAGERS AND POLICYMAKERS

Thomas G. Rundall, Peter F. Martelli, Rodney McCurdy, Ilana Graetz, Laura Arroyo, Esther B. Neuwirth, Pam Curtis, Julie Schmittdiel, Mark Gibson, and John Hsu

Introduction

Using research evidence when making decisions about the organization, financing, and delivery of healthcare has great appeal, yet research suggests that health services managers routinely do not consider it. One observer described health services researchers and practitioners as "strangers in the night, dimly aware of each other's presence" (Lomas 2000). Innovative organizations that do use research evidence to support their decisions may take years, if not decades, to disseminate this information. This gap between the collection and use of evidence is a serious concern, because important decisions may not benefit from the best available information. Moreover, health services research has limited societal value if rarely used.

Managers eschew research evidence in their decision making for many reasons. It may not be timely or relevant to their priorities; the findings may be poorly communicated; the evidence may draw on contextually ignorant or irrelevant studies; or the findings may not suggest actionable steps. For some decisions, high-quality, useful evidence may not exist. Moreover, decision makers may have varying requirements with respect to the amount, type, or definition of evidence they need. To understand better the reasons for this gap between evidence and practice and to identify possible remedies, we convened peer-to-peer focus groups of senior health services managers and policymakers to discuss their views about using research evidence in decision making.

How the Research Was Conducted

Study Sample and Data Collection

We convened four peer-to-peer, full-day focus groups with 32 senior decision makers from 26 public and private organizations from eastern, midwestern, and western regions of the United States. Focus groups are an efficient way to collect detailed information about complex social processes, including initial responses and reactions to viewpoints expressed by other participants. During the focus group sessions, participants responded to questions about:

- Types of high-priority strategic decisions facing their organizations;
- Current use of research evidence in managerial and policy decision making;
- Characteristics of useful evidence;
- Organizational barriers to using evidence; and
- Suggestions for increasing the use of evidence in decision making.

We used purposive sampling to recruit participants for the focus groups. To incorporate the needs of a wide range of organizations, we invited managers (typically directors, chief operating officers, and chief executive officers) from the public and private sectors, including hospitals, physician practices, health maintenance organizations, health insurance companies, Medicaid programs, and regulatory agencies. Moreover, we included some managers from organizations that have limited resources. Thirty-two managers accepted our invitation, resulting in focus groups within our target size of five to ten persons, representing varied organization types.

Focus groups were conducted in San Francisco (test); Oakland, California; Chicago; and New York City. Participants attended an introduction and overview dinner the evening before the sessions. The meetings lasted seven hours, with a working lunch. To provide an environment that encouraged open and candid discussions, we guaranteed the participants' confidentiality.

One of our investigators presented instructions about the focus group process; another moderated, took whiteboard notes, directed the conversation, prompted participants to elaborate on relevant topics, and periodically summarized the conversation. At least two researchers took notes during the meeting—one aiming to produce a transcript-like document, and the other focusing on themes and notable quotations. We were free to interact with the participants, but we focused that interaction on clarification so we would not overly influence the course of the discussion.

After the initial test group, discussions were divided into three sections:

- Descriptions of participants' organizations, their perspective on the availability and use of management evidence, and an example of using or not using evidence in the organization's decision-making process;
- A brainstorming session, organized around the type, format, and rigor of useful evidence, and the skills, tools, and organizational capabilities required to use evidence; and

Box 1.1
Thematic
Categories
Used in Initial
Coding of
Focus Group
Discussions

I. Framework for Decisions
   a. Types of decisions
   b. Examples of using or not using research evidence during
       specific decisions
   c. Decision-making time frames

II. Characteristics of Useful Evidence
   a. Evidence definitions
   b. Sources of evidence
   c. Characteristics of evidence
   d. Criteria for evaluating evidence
   e. Examples of weighing different sources or characteristics
       of information

III. Organizational Barriers to and Facilitators of Using Evidence
   a. Factors (e.g., skills, structures, resources, and capabilities)
       perceived to be needed
   b. Factors currently available
   c. Barriers

IV. Communication/Collaboration to Link and Exchange Information
   a. Methods, tactics, or barriers for decision makers to articulate
       their evidence needs
   b. Methods, channels, and media for producers of evidence to
       communicate evidence
   c. Methods, tactics, or barriers for collaborating with researchers

V. Suggestions for an Evidence-Based Management Toolbox
   a. Characteristics of a useful toolbox

- A review of the session's notes, refinement of those notes, and a closing report. Major themes—such as definitions of evidence, organizational management, and policy priorities—and barriers to the use of evidence were fine-tuned in this section.

Data Analysis

We analyzed each focus group transcript in three steps. First, we reviewed the transcripts and developed a refined coding protocol. Second, two researchers read each transcript and coded participants' comments into 15 predetermined thematic categories central to our understanding of managers' and policymakers' use of research evidence (Box 1.1). The researchers initially agreed on 74 percent of the coded statements, then discussed the others and reached consensus. Third, we analyzed the content of comments in each of the thematic categories.

What We Learned

Types of Strategic Decisions

From the focus group participants' discussion, we identified five broad types of high-priority strategic decisions and specific categories of decisions within each type (Box 1.2).

The most frequently mentioned decisions involved the purchase of products or systems to improve quality and reduce costs—for example, pharmaceuticals (which are particularly important for Medicaid agencies), information technology, and medical technology. Other high-priority decisions included finding methods to improve the organization and delivery of care, particularly care for patients with chronic diseases, and improving quality, increasing patient safety, and reducing the cost of care.

Another set of decisions clustered around the theme of organizational sustainability: strategic planning, change management, managing decision making in multi-institutional organizations, leadership development, managing the delivery organization's physician strategy, and generally improving organizational performance. These issues relate to the decisions organizations must make to adapt to changing environments, develop internal leadership, and maintain effective relationships with a key strategic partner—physicians.

Managers of health plans emphasized the importance of plan benefit design and coverage decisions in their work, whereas managers of delivery organizations emphasized the importance of workforce recruitment, development, and retention.

Use of Research Evidence in the Decision-Making Process

Participants reported little use of research evidence in policymaking or managerial decision making. Several participants expressed general familiarity with evidence-based *medicine*, which focuses on care of a particular patient; fewer participants were familiar with evidence-based *management* or *policymaking*, which focuses on the support of high-performance care. Comments reflecting this confusion include:

> *We're looking to those major organizations [NCQA, Joint Commission, National Quality Forum] and those major specialty societies, like the American College of Cardiology, for guidelines. But, there just aren't enough guidelines out there to evaluate physician practices.*

> *It gets at the basic issue of what will clinicians listen to, whom will they listen to? They're not going to listen to a health insurer. They're not going to listen to the feds in all likelihood, except as much as they can twist their arm. The credible sources for clinicians, I think, are their professional societies.*

Box 1.2
Types of
Strategic
Decisions
Participants
Made

Healthcare Purchasing (46 mentions)
> Cost-effective purchasing of healthcare products and services (36)
> Information technology purchase and implementation (6)
> Technology assessment (4)

Organization and Delivery of Patient Care (22 mentions)
> Chronic disease management (11)
> Providing incentives to patients/changing behaviors (2)
> Redesign for patient safety (2)
> Patient satisfaction (2)
> Moving care to post-hospital settings (1)
> Use of hospitalists (1)
> Developing quality indicators (1)
> Utilization of pain management tools (1)
> Ambulatory visit scheduling/redesign (1)

Strategic Positioning/Management (17 mentions)
> Strategic market analysis (5)
> Implementation and change management (3)
> Local versus group/system decision making (3)
> Leadership development/succession planning (2)
> Physician strategy management (2)
> Organizational performance (2)

Benefit Design/Coverage Decisions/Product Design (10 mentions)
> Medicaid design (6)
> Universal healthcare (2)
> Patient copays (1)
> Managed care for the aged, blind, and disabled (1)

Workforce Recruitment, Development, and Retention (10 mentions)
> Staffing roles, responsibilities, and workforce development (7)
> Physician satisfaction (1)
> Benefits to retirees (1)
> Employee health promotion/disease prevention (1)

And some of these nonprofit entities like the National Quality Forum that vet this information.

What I want for clinical decision making is randomized controlled trials. That's the standard. If I can get that, and it points to a certain direction, then that means it supports a particular therapy or is against a particular therapy or intervention. It's hard to base large-scale clinical changes on anything less than that.

But even when the idea of using research evidence to help managers and policymakers make decisions about organizational issues was clarified, only one participant in all of the sessions stated that such an approach was routinely used in his organization. Interestingly, some respondents indicated they believed they did use evidence, but their definition of evidence differed from that typically used by researchers.

Definitions of Evidence

The participants defined *evidence* broadly and included information beyond that gained from empirical scientific studies (Box 1.3). They agreed that scientific information on causal relationships was evidence, but they also defined evidence as personal experience, advice from peers, recommendations from vendors, policies and regulations pertaining to a decision, and reports from other organizations. Particularly valuable, according to several participants, was information from pilot studies of organizational changes, case studies of managerial decisions in other organizations, and qualitative assessments of operational or strategic decisions by peers or acknowledged experts.

Several participants noted that they believe managers used such a range of information because of the trust they have in personal experience, the difficulty in translating research evidence into practice, and the unsuitability of most research evidence to meet their decision-making needs. As one participant said:

We have people who have been there 20-plus years and so we have tacit knowledge—we are very successful—in our experience, success brings success.

Another participant said that, with the existing scientific literature:

There's no way to reach conclusions.

Still another said:

Very little evidence [on the management side] is used in the classical sense, but what are necessary are dashboard items. And every manager needs evidence that's documented, but it's a different sort. You need employment-related information, you need rate information, you need competitive information, you need a lot of market-based information that doesn't meet the [scientific] rigor, but still is vital information for managers.

Sources of Evidence

Given these health managers' and policymakers' broad definition of evidence, it is not surprising that participants reported a wide range of evidence sources (Box 1.4). The range also reflects the fragmented and disorganized knowledge environment in which managers make decisions. In the absence of a recognized lead external organization or internal research capacity, managers

Box 1.3
How
Participants
Defined
Evidence

Internal Data/Measurements (5 mentions)
- Readmission rates, complications, and mortality (2)
- Payment rates (1)
- Cost (1)
- Employment information (1)

Colloquial Evidence (2 mentions)
- Information from vendors (1)
- Experiences of respected organizations (e.g., best practices from another organization) (1)

Scientific Evidence (i.e., information demonstrating causal relationships) (1 mention)
- Controlled studies (1)

Externally Dictated Standards (1 mention)
- Applicable regulations (e.g., defining medical necessity) (1)

Narratives (meeting summary boards) (1 mention)

Box 1.4
Sources of
Evidence

Validating Organizations/External Standards (39 mentions)
- Examples: Agency for Healthcare Research and Quality, National Committee for Quality Assurance, National Quality Forum, The Cochrane Collaboration, American College of Cardiology, California HealthCare Foundation, Institute for Healthcare Improvement, Institute of Medicine

Knowledge Brokers/Experts (11 mentions)
- Examples: Consultants, peers with comparable experience, academic experts

Advocates (10 mentions)
- Examples: Vendors, advocacy groups

Conferences/Professional Exchanges (9 mentions)
- Examples: Oregon HSC Drug Effectiveness Project, roundtables

Databases/Internal Feedback (9 mentions)
- Examples: Internal system reports, environmental scans

Information from the Internet/Media (7 mentions)
- Examples: Google, newspapers

Regulations/Case Law (2 mentions)
- Examples: Case law, state government requirements

Literature—Written (1 mention)
- Example: *New England Journal of Medicine*

often look for information from any source they can readily locate. The quality of these sources varies with each individual decision maker's experiences, skills, and network of contacts.

Of 88 total mentions of sources of evidence, only one participant mentioned print journals as a source of evidence, and that was the *New England Journal of Medicine*. Participants reported that they rarely read traditional research journals. Two quotes from different participants capture the opinions expressed by many others:

> *We bring together roundtables to see what is working—may not be scientific, but we get a lot of information that way. We often see where we are not doing enough as well.*

> *We use evidence in the deployment of key strategic decisions. We'll use books, vendors, best practices, to the extent that there's literature available. Not sure if it qualifies as evidence, but then, we haven't defined what evidence is.*

Useful and Relevant Evidence: Criteria for Evaluation

Despite the wide range of information that participants considered useful and relevant, they agreed that it should meet four basic criteria (Box 1.5): accuracy, applicability, actionability, and accessibility. For example, they wanted evidence that provides a complete picture—the "good, bad, and ugly." They were more concerned about accuracy than precision: As one manager said, "I do not think that management decisions [need to be] 95 percent [in terms of certainty]. I would be happy with 70 to 80 percent."

Two comments reveal the anxiety participants experience in evaluating the quality and usefulness of evidence and their desire for help from others, perhaps governmental organizations, in determing these features:

> *There's an issue of transparency—both in the evidence and in the way it is gathered. Most people don't have the resources to do this [evaluate evidence] on their own.*

> *If there is a nationally recognized process that's transparent where the state can have its own committee come in and review it and maybe tweak it, it becomes completely transparent, and I think you're more likely to succeed at the local level.*

Perceived Barriers to Use of Evidence-Based Management

Factors in the larger healthcare environment, as well as local circumstances, can be barriers to using research information (Box 1.6). Environmental

Box 1.5
Criteria Used
to Evaluate
Evidence

Is the Information Accurate?
- Is the source credible, including having unbiased support?
- Does it establish a causal relationship?
- Does it provide a complete, balanced viewpoint?
- Does the presentation provide information on the relevant statistical properties, without eliminating data based on arbitrary standards of precision?
- Does it provide adequate information on the limitations?
- Is the process transparent?

Is the Information Applicable to My Decision?
- Does it apply to my organization, market, and situation?
- Does it state when it is applicable and when it is not?

Does the Information Include Actionable Steps?
- Does it describe what needs to be done?
- Does the availability of the information fit into the time frame of my decision?
- Does it provide a complete set of implications, including costs?
- Does it include consideration of the overall decision context, including other available information?

Is the Relevant Information Accessible?
- Is it easy to obtain when I need it?
- Is the presentation easy to digest, without having to work to find the relevant items?

barriers to the use of evidence, such as state or federal laws regulating personnel policies, typically require a substantial effort to change and are often beyond the influence of any single organization. Local barriers, such as weak organizational leadership support, are largely under the control of individual organizations.

Participants cited organizational culture as a barrier more often than any other factor. Other frequently mentioned barriers were inadequate resources; the difficulty of doing evidence-based management (EB management); lack of knowledge about EB management; restrictions on decision making due to human resource policies, regulations, laws, etc.; political and institutional pressures; and weak leadership support.

Of special interest to the management and policy research communities is the finding that 8 of the 28 mentions of environmental barriers indicated that *inadequate methods or evidence* was a barrier to use of research evidence:

For the vast majority of questions I have, I have found the answers are not out there. Research is not being done in a way that answers my questions.

Box 1.6
Barriers to Use
of Evidence-
Based
Management

Environmental (28 mentions)
- Restrictions on decisions linked to human resource policies, regulations, case law, etc. (13)
- Political and institutional environment (7)
  ○ Political advocacy, politics (5)
  ○ External environment not supportive of evidence-based management (1)
  ○ Proprietary interests (1)
- Inadequate methods or evidence (8)
  ○ Evidence that is weak, unclear, conflicting, unconvincing (6)
  ○ Lack of transparency in methods/evidence (1)
  ○ Lack of evidence on the use of evidence in making decisions (1)

Local (93 mentions)
- Culture (values, beliefs, priorities) (26)
- Resources (money, time, technology, data) (23)
- Difficulty of applying evidence-based management (20)
  ○ Difficulty of accessing, appraising, applying evidence (10)
  ○ Takes too long (7)
  ○ Too much variation in management questions and context (2)
  ○ Medicaid chronic disease population that is hard to capture (1)
- Lack of knowledge about evidence-based management (14)
- Weak organizational leadership support (8)
  ○ Leadership that is weak, turns over, is not supportive (4)
  ○ Consultants used instead of evidence-based management (4)
- Difficulty of measuring outcomes of decisions based on evidence (1)
- Lack of formal organizational structure for the application of evidence (1)

Factors Perceived to Be Needed to Use Evidence

Participants said numerous factors are necessary for the systematic use of evidence in organizational decision making (Box 1.7). Most frequently mentioned was the development and support of EB management by a respected national organization. Respondents believed such an organization could provide a foundation for the improvement of EB management by working systematically with providers, health plans, and other organizations; increase access to useful evidence; legitimatize the practice of EB management; and certify evidence judged to meet some minimal standards.

Other factors considered important to this effort included supportive leadership at all levels, education and skill development in EB management, more and better evidence, and the creation and dissemination of tools to help managers use evidence in decision making.

Box 1.7
Factors
Perceived to
Be Needed to
Increase Use
of Evidence

Environmental (37 mentions)
- National, respected organization to develop and support evidence-based management (11)
- Clearinghouse for management evidence (7)
- More and better evidence (6)
- Communication and dissemination tools (post to a blog, expert contacts, clinical participation) (3)
- Evidence on change and organizational behavior (3)
- Indication of evidence's legitimacy (2)
- More studies (general) (2)
- Common criteria (2)
- Partnerships with university programs (1)

Local (53 mentions)
- Leadership at local, state, and federal levels (10)
- Education about evidence-based management (10)
- Tools that facilitate evidence search and collection (10)
- Resources (time, money, etc.) (7)
- Structures for integrating evidence into work processes (7)
- Cultural change (e.g., more accountability, value attached to evidence) (7)
- Dashboard items (1)
- Incentives (1)

Participants also identified a need for more internal organizational resources (time and money) to perform the work required to do EB management, new structures and processes (committees, task forces, webmasters, specialized staff, etc.), cultural changes, communication and dissemination tools, incentives, and partnerships with knowledge brokers and evidence producers.

Implications of the Findings

Two major points summarize our key findings:

1. Decision makers report using research evidence rarely; instead, they rely on recommendations from external organizations, personal experience, and the experiences of peers and consultants.
2. Decision makers perceive that the content and accessibility of existing research are inadequate.

These findings are consistent with other studies conducted in the United States, Canada, and the United Kingdom (Canadian Health Services Research Foundation 2000, 2004; Lavis et al. 2002; Kovner and Rundall 2006). They contribute to a substantial body of research documenting the gap between health services research and management/policymaking communities. Our findings clarify the reasons for this gap and point to a number of actions that could reduce it.

Health services researchers must be trained and retrained to conduct and communicate research in ways that increase the likelihood health services managers and policymakers will use it. Our study demonstrated that useful, practice-oriented research evidence must have what we call the four As—*accuracy, applicability, actionability*, and *accessibility*. Managers and policymakers believe that useful evidence must provide a complete and balanced viewpoint from a credible source (i.e., be accurate); be relevant to the management question of interest (i.e., be applicable); include information on what needs to be done and likely implications (i.e., be actionable); and be easy to obtain and understand (i.e., be accessible).

Our study participants understood that researchers typically believe that they cannot generalize study evidence and resulting recommendations beyond a fairly narrow set of circumstances, including the type of population studied, the nature of the organizations included, and the characteristics of the policy and regulatory environments in which the studied organizations functioned. Evidence that emerges from a study that does not fit those circumstances is unlikely to be used. Finally, the evidence and its presentation should incorporate an assessment of the confidence researchers have in the validity of the findings, and the link between the study findings and specific recommendations should be clear.

A brief, carefully structured synopsis of the research, such as the *plain language summaries* attached to the research syntheses prepared by the Effective Practice and Organization of Care branch of the Cochrane Collaboration (www.cochrane.org/reviews/en/topics/61.html), will likely increase the use of a study's findings.

Collaborative relationships between health services researchers and practitioners need to be encouraged and supported. Some advocacy is already under way, such as the Agency for Healthcare Research and Quality's (AHRQ) Accelerating Change and Transformation in Organizations and Networks (ACTION) program, the work of the Health Research and Educational Trust's Center for Health Management Research, and the American Health Insurance Plans' annual Building Bridges Conference. Still, these efforts touch only a fraction of the health services research, management, and policy communities, and they should be expanded.

We agree with the recent call for a national evidence-based healthcare management center or program (Shortell 2006) that could be carried out by the AHRQ and monitored by the National Quality Forum and related groups. The primary responsibilities of this entity would be to ensure that relevant management and organizational research is rigorously assessed, to encourage more meta-analyses, to make reliable evidence in a usable form widely available to managers and policymakers, and to help link such evidence to decision-making processes in health services organizations.[1]

Our findings also suggest a number of actions leaders of health services organizations can take to help bridge the gap between management research, policy research, and practice. The most important step is to build organizational cultures, processes, and structures that support the use of research evidence in decision making. Here are some possible actions health-care managers can take:

- Implement systematic processes for making major decisions.
- Periodically brief managers on recent research related to the organization's operational and strategic concerns.
- Incorporate research assessments into due diligence reports.
- Train management team members in the steps of evidence-based decision making.
- Establish ties with academic institutions and research centers.

The latter step would enable linkage and exchange among researchers, managers, and policymakers. It would not only increase the use of evidence in decision making, but also provide opportunities for the practice community to constructively influence the research performed by health services researchers.

Endnote

1. Examples of similar organizations include the NHS Service Delivery and Organisation Programme (http://www.sdo.lshtm.ac.uk/) in the United Kingdom and the Canadian Health Services Research Foundation (http://www.chsrf.ca).

References

Canadian Health Services Research Foundation. 2000. *Health Services Research and Evidence-based Decision Making, 7*. Ottawa, Canada.

_____ 2004. *What Counts? Interpreting Evidence-based Decision-making for Management and Policy*. Ottawa, Canada.

Kovner, A. R., and T. G. Rundall. 2006. "Evidence-based Management Reconsidered." *Frontiers of Health Services Management* 22: 3–22.

Lavis, J. N., S. E. Ross, J. E. Hurley, J. M. Hohenadel, G. L. Stoddart, C. A. Woodward, and J. Abelson. 2002. "Examining the Role of Health Services Research in Public Policy Making." *Milbank Quarterly* 80: 125–53.

Lomas, J. 2000. "Using 'Linkage and Exchange' to Move Research Into Policy at a Canadian Foundation." *Health Affairs* 19: 236–40.

Shortell, S. M. 2006. "Promoting Evidence-Based Management." *Frontiers of Health Services Management* 22: 23–29.

APPLICATION OF EVIDENCE-BASED MANAGEMENT AT AN ACADEMIC MEDICAL CENTER: THE YALE-NEW HAVEN HOSPITAL EXPERIENCE

Richard D'Aquila

Introduction

This chapter describes a comprehensive and contemporary movement toward evidence-based management (EB management) at a large academic medical center. It profiles a model for incorporating evidence-based analysis and decision making in all major dimensions of organizational performance, including strategic planning, resource allocation, quality and safety surveillance, performance management, and operational dashboard systems designed to provide real-time assessments.

This chapter demonstrates that an EB management approach enables managers in healthcare organizations to elevate the performance of their institutions—and their own effectiveness as leaders—by improving the quality of their decisions. It illustrates how EB management can be at the core of a set of principles and behaviors guiding efforts to continuously improve hospital performance.

For EB management to work, organizations must:

- Make comprehensive performance information systems visible and available to the entire staff;
- Strategize planning and decision making regarding major resource investments;
- Perform evaluations of, and offer rewards for, leaders' performance; and
- Have a method of monitoring their "vital signs" and deciding where to channel problem-solving efforts.

In short, EB management is the underpinning of a culture that demands discipline, rewards performance, and encourages a climate that has little tolerance for the status quo. The next section describes our experience at Yale-New Haven Hospital in New Haven, Connecticut, which has incorporated EB management principles in every facet of organizational performance.

About Yale-New Haven Hospital

The nation's fourth hospital—originally chartered in 1826—Yale-New Haven Hospital (YNHH) is the largest and most comprehensive hospital in Connecticut. It is a 944-licensed-bed tertiary referral center that includes 270 beds designated as the Yale-New Haven Children's Hospital and 72 beds in the nearby Yale-New Haven Psychiatric Hospital.

YNHH is the primary teaching hospital for the Yale University School of Medicine (YSM) and is one of 50 teaching hospitals nationwide that together train nearly 40 percent of all U.S. medical residents.

Evidence-Based Management: Application of Principles at Yale-New Haven Hospital

The following applications of EB management illustrate YNHH's comprehensive approach, which integrates strategic planning, performance monitoring, management objectives, and operating dashboards.

Service Line Planning

One of the major challenges facing executives in an academic medical center is making informed decisions about growth management, service expansion, and investments. With hospital beds, staff, and available capital in short supply, administrators must make intelligent, data-driven decisions about the allocation of these resources. Academic medical centers have additional pressures to develop and maintain clinical and research programs that attract top national talent and build clinical excellence on a regional and national basis.

YNHH has adopted service line planning as its model for making these critical resource allocation decisions and achieving consensus on strategic direction. YSM also has adopted this process to ensure that the hospital and university are jointly planning for clinical program development that reflects sound investment decisions.

Service line planning, patterned on product lines in manufacturing, is not a new model in healthcare. Since the 1980s, hospitals across the country have recognized the value of developing strategic plans according to discrete clinical business categories. YNHH studied the attempts of others to adopt service line planning and modified the model to accommodate the particular attributes of the hospital and university. The structure of YNHH is a matrix. Some managers (called clinical service coordinators) have specific service responsibilities (for oncology or pediatrics, for example), and some managers have traditional line-management responsibilities. YNHH created the matrix largely to support the service line model.

YNHH selects operational improvement initiatives according to priorities it establishes annually in its business plan. It closely monitors operational performance through a set of indicators and identifies improvement opportunities when these indicators begin to lag. An operations group, comprising the vice presidents, senior vice presidents, and executive vice presidents, meets weekly to review the indicators and determine whether action is required. This model of regular, high-level performance monitoring is replicated throughout the organization—down to the unit level.

Prior to adopting the service line model, YNHH had a more traditional planning process that did not directly engage the school of medicine. The process was largely opportunistic and not helpful in establishing priorities for growth. Using service line planning, YNHH has been able to:

- Conduct realistic assessments of its current position;
- Set a clear vision and road map;
- Create a sense of discomfort with the status quo;
- Communicate vision and priorities in multiple forums, led by a vocal and visible leadership group;
- Align the organizational structure with strategic priorities (i.e., the service lines); and
- Constantly reinforce key messages through initiatives and funding decisions.

The cost of service line planning is difficult to quantify. However, for the initial five service lines, over the first six months of fiscal year 2007, the Planning Department spent approximately 2,700 hours on all aspects of the service line initiative, including data formulation, data runs, analysis, review, and meetings. As YNHH is still in the recommendation phases for several of these service lines, management cannot yet estimate the full cost associated with the implementation.

Principles and Organization

Service line planning at YNHH enables management to develop comprehensive strategic plans for delivering a continuum of services for each major clinical service group. The process enables maximum physician input. Select committees lead the overall effort and planning for the five initial service lines (Figure 2.1).

The five initial service lines are:

- **Transplant Service Line:** kidney, pancreas, liver, small bowel
- **Neuroscience Service Line:** neurology, neurosurgery, stroke, spine, interventional neuroradiology, brain and spine trauma, brain cancer
- **Cardiovascular Service Line:** cardiac surgery, cardiology, vascular surgery imaging, cardiac and lung transplant, endovascular, electrophysiology

FIGURE 2.1
Service Line
Planning
Structure

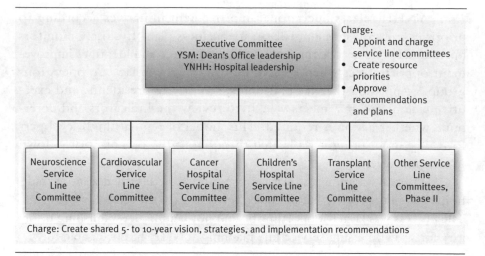

Charge: Create shared 5- to 10-year vision, strategies, and implementation recommendations

- **Cancer Service Line:** all screening, diagnostic, and treatment services for patients with known or suspected neoplasms
- **Children's Service Line:** Inpatient services and ambulatory services for patients (1) registered with a children's hospital for care; (2) whose physician is from the Department of Pediatrics, the pediatric section of another department (e.g., Pediatric Surgery), or a known pediatric provider in a non-pediatric area (e.g., pediatric trauma surgeon, neurosurgeon); and (3) under age 18, regardless of location or physician.

Also, management tentatively identified seven additional service lines for subsequent planning efforts:

- Behavioral Health
- Women's Services
- Gastrointestinal Disease
- Vascular Disease
- Geriatrics
- Emergency/Ambulatory Care
- Orthopedics

The Executive Committee, which has joint and equal representation by YSM and YNHH senior leadership teams, governs the overall process. It meets monthly, appoints and sets the charge for each service line committee, and reviews all interim findings. More important, the Executive Committee reviews all strategic and programmatic recommendations and gives final approval of all resource recommendations, priorities, and commitments.

Use of the Evidence-Based Management Approach

Step 1. Framing the Question. The planning team identified 12 to 13 potential service lines from observation of how patients cluster around various clinical services. From this list, it selected the first group of service lines by determining which of the services have the greatest impact—especially financial—on the hospital, and which face possible increase or decrease due to various internal and external forces.

Step 2. Finding Information. The team conducted extensive research, following a standardized format for data collection. Project teams focused on identifying best practices, collecting and reviewing relevant industry and market-specific data, and employing other forms of data collection and analysis.

Step 3. Evaluating the Information. The team drew on the standard data set for each service line and conducted SWOT (strengths/weaknesses/opportunities/threats) and other types of analyses. A committee with broad representation from key clinical and administrative leadership evaluated this information.

Step 4. Applicability and Actionability of the Information. Determination of applicability involved facilitated discussion and decision making. Using the children's service line as an example, the planning group developed specific recommendations regarding vision and strategic focus, physician recruitment priorities, geographic deployment, and program growth. It shared these recommendations with the Dean's Office and the YNHH President's Office to obtain their consent.

Step 5. Adequacy of the Information. Management concluded that the information used to discuss the service lines' priorities provided sufficient detail and balance to draw reasonable conclusions.

Work Product and Process

Building a service line plan is a disciplined and data-driven process at YNHH. Each service line committee includes a trained facilitator, supported by finance staff and planning and information specialists from the hospital and university. Committees range from 16 to 25 members, approximately equally divided between physicians and hospital managers, and are co-chaired by a representative of management from YNHH and a clinical chief from YSM. Committees emphasize creating a common and thorough understanding of the marketplace; emerging trends in technology and treatment; and strengths, weaknesses, and market position of the service. In some service lines, such as children's and cancer treatment, national benchmarks exist, as do data on strategic characteristics of competitive facilities like Boston Children's Hospital and Memorial Sloan-Kettering Cancer Center.

Figure 2.2 displays the schedule for a typical committee and the progression from strategic situational assessment to the development of

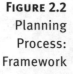

FIGURE 2.2
Planning
Process:
Framework

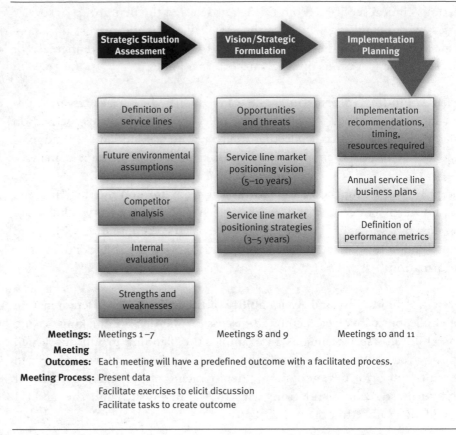

implementation plans. As this process is highly structured and involves assimilation of considerable amounts of data, trained facilitators and polished data presentations are essential to maintaining a project schedule.

Key elements of committees' plans include:

1. A current assessment of the service line (SWOT analysis) supported by:
   • market share and volume trend information (inpatient and outpatient, if available)
   • current out-migration data from the New Haven area and from YNHH to other hospitals
   • national utilization estimates
   • payer-mix data
   • existing complement of beds and physicians
   • upstream/downstream linkages
   • service issues (e.g., from Press-Ganey patient satisfaction surveys, employee opinion surveys, and physician surveys)

2. Development of a 5- to 10-year vision for the service

3. Requirements and factors critical to achieving the vision, including:
   • organizational structure requirements (clinical and administrative)

- market strategies to address national and local trends
- physician recruitment strategies with supporting financial plans
- technology and capital requirements with supporting financial plans
- a financial plan for the service line
- fundraising development strategies (as appropriate)

4. Action steps and strategies for achieving the vision

5. Metrics to monitor and assess performance, such as market share growth relative to competition, percentile rankings for treatment complications and mortality, opportunities to fulfill unmet community needs within the service line, and patient/physician/employee satisfaction targets

6. Time frames and accountability assignments, such as:
   - What steps will we take now versus two years from now?
   - Which parties will be responsible?
   - What will the process and deadlines be?

The committees' work sets a vision and strategy for each service line, which ultimately drive specific implementation recommendations. Once approved by the Executive Committee, these recommendations find their way into physician recruitment efforts, annual service line plans, and, in some cases, ongoing performance measures, such as service utilization targets. Figure 2.3 depicts this transition from service line planning to operational priorities.

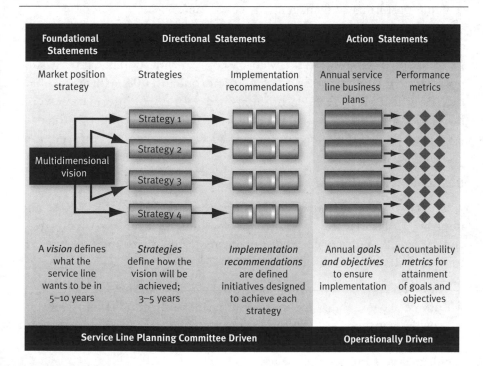

FIGURE 2.3
Strategic Template

Conclusions

Service line planning has proved to be a valuable application of EB management at YNHH. As a strategic planning process, it already has:

- Created a common clinical vision in high-priority service lines;
- Supported decisions around programs, people, facilities, and the allocation of limited resources in a manner that best supports the common vision;
- Positioned key clinical services to gain and maintain regional, national, and international stature;
- Set the foundation for realignment of the hospital's leadership, in particular the assignment of key senior leadership positions to major service lines; and
- Established productive partnerships between the hospital and YSM.

Performance Management Information Technology

YNHH was the driving force behind the development of Yale New Haven Health System (YNHHS) in 1991. The four-hospital system spans coastal Connecticut and eastern Rhode Island, and includes YNHH, Greenwich Hospital (Greenwich, Connecticut), Bridgeport Hospital (Bridgeport, Connecticut), and Westerly Hospital (Westerly, Rhode Island). This system's founding principles included a commitment to endeavors that would have system-wide strategic value, such as deployment of information system and performance management technologies.

Development of a YNHHS performance management system was an early goal. Ultimately called PMIT—Performance Management Information Technology—this web-based, real-time system centrally supports three major databases containing more than 100 performance metrics. Prior to PMIT, YNHHS hospitals had a variety of information storehouses in different locations, which compromised the validity of the data (as sources and definitions conflicted) and timely access to information.

Design and Function

The performance management initiative was designed to evaluate and improve YNHHS's ability to provide the highest level of patient safety, clinical quality, and service, while enhancing productivity and financial performance. Its objectives were to:

- Translate YNHHS business plans into clear, measurable outcomes;
- Enforce accountability for successful business plan implementation;
- Provide managers and clinical leaders with the training, education, and resources they need to continuously monitor, communicate, analyze, and enhance performance;

- Drive cross-functional collaboration and sharing of best practices; and
- Provide quantitative evidence of YNHHS accomplishments.

Another performance management goal was to "flatten" the organization by:

- Increasing its limited access to enterprise information to broad access through PMIT and the information portal;
- Moving from an organization where only some managers have the required training and improvement tools to one in which all managers have access to these resources; and
- Bridging the disconnect between corporate objectives and improvement initiatives so that improvement expertise is focused on significant problems.

The performance management initiative is led by the vice president of performance management, who reports to the executive vice president of strategy and system development, and who is supported by a performance management director and resource group that includes Six Sigma–trained individuals at each YNHHS hospital. The System Executive Committee oversaw the development and implementation of the performance management initiative and recommended which PMIT reports would be created, distributed, or discontinued.

A key deliverable of the performance management initiative is the PMIT Balanced Scorecard, the value of which depends on how effectively the information influences decisions that improve performance. The Balanced Scorecard reflects real-time information systems organized and designed to support the four broad categories of annual business plans for the system as a whole and for YNHH, as follows:

- Patient safety, quality, and operations improvement
- Provider of choice
- Employer of choice
- Financial performance

Thus, the PMIT system supports the business plans and objectives on which the hospital and system base their annual performance assessment.

As of December 2006, three PMIT scorecards were live—an executive scorecard that has 30 metrics, an operating room scorecard that has 18 metrics (with an additional 12 under development), and a clinical quality scorecard that has 42 metrics. The following reports are regularly updated on the PMIT website:

- Inpatient activity
- Census variance
- Daily census, discharges
- Vacancy rate

- Intensive Care Unit quality
- Surgical infection rates
- Case management

Performance outcomes to date, in areas such as ICU services, indicate significant positive improvements, several of which were highlighted in the introduction to this chapter.

Challenges and Next Steps

YNHHS was an early adopter of comprehensive, system-wide performance information systems. The system has a strong analytical capacity, features distinctive graphical presentation, and is available on every management desktop.

Despite being over a decade old, this initiative is regarded as a work in progress and is subject to continuous investment and improvement. The system has confronted several ongoing challenges in its continued evolution, particularly the need to standardize definitions and data structures across hospitals and to ensure the integrity and timeliness of data, even as primary data sources change. Nevertheless, PMIT is considered a valuable system-wide management support tool that has enabled leadership to establish accountability and has given managers the information they need to make better decisions.

YNHH continues to drive performance expectations down to the department and unit levels in an attempt to enable all managers to lead their business units with the influence and authority of a CEO. Each manager is held accountable, both generally and specifically, for (in most cases) seven dimensions of performance:

- Volume, flow, and throughput
- Financial performance (profit and loss or expense management)
- Quality of care
- Regulatory and accreditation readiness
- Patient/customer satisfaction
- Employee satisfaction
- Medical staff satisfaction

Achieving the Corporate Objectives

Explicit corporate objectives are critical communication and motivational tools. One way to assess performance is to make each employee responsible for achieving these objectives as they apply to his or her role.

Where assessment based on a peer group or best practice is appropriate, management typically compares its hospital's performance against organizations with similar missions and demographics (size, scope of services, payer mix, patient acuity, etc.). Where a regional comparison is desirable, such as vacancy rates, performance is usually benchmarked against other local hospitals. For still other metrics—most often financial and efficiency measures—performance may be measured against that of other industries.

Summary and Conclusion

This chapter demonstrated several applications of EB management that dramatically improved managers' ability to elevate the performance of their areas of responsibility and the institution as a whole. The case examples illustrate an organizational philosophy and process based on inquiry, data-driven decisions, and performance excellence. In its commitment to consistent performance improvement, hospital leadership continues its efforts to enhance the application and use of evidence-based decision making with each new challenge and opportunity.

EVIDENCE-BASED MANAGEMENT AS A TRANSFORMATIONAL LEVER AT ST. LUKE'S EPISCOPAL HEALTH SYSTEM

David J. Fine and Emily L. Garrison

Introduction

St. Luke's Episcopal Hospital was founded in 1954 with a $1 million gift from Hugh Roy Cullen that paralleled contributions made in the same amount to the Methodist and Baptist churches—all for the purpose of founding new hospitals in what would later become the Texas Medical Center. Initial construction at St. Luke's resulted in twin pavilions with shared ancillary services for 130 adult and 106 pediatric beds. Pediatric programs were reorganized into the independent Texas Children's Hospital in 1987. Licensed adult capacity peaked at 948 adult beds in 2001. By 2004, average daily adult census was 525, with capacity of 719 operational beds.

A new CEO was recruited to join the St. Luke's Episcopal Health System effective June 14, 2004.

Initial Assessment

The new CEO began his engagement by spending the first two months in a "deep listening" process to independently ascertain strengths, weaknesses, opportunities, and threats associated with the various business units and critical stakeholders that make up St. Luke's. The CEO reported the results of this activity at a special meeting of the board of directors in late August 2004. The preliminary picture was not comforting.

In general, St. Luke's enjoyed a favorable public reputation, as evidenced by its stature as an employer of choice in greater Houston and multiyear recognition as one of *Fortune* magazine's "100 Best Employers" (2002, 2004, and 2005), along with such popular exemplars as Microsoft, Proctor & Gamble, General Mills, and Starbucks. *U.S. News & World Report* listed the Texas Heart Institute at St. Luke's Episcopal Hospital among the top 10 cardiovascular centers of excellence in the United States for 17 consecutive years (1991–2007). Further, the health system enjoyed a Standard & Poor's credit rating for 2004 of "AA–," a recognition accorded to less than 14 percent of all independently rated U.S. hospitals that year.

Hospital employees were proud of this recognition. However, comparison of organizational and operational fundamentals with those of similar hospitals and health systems revealed many opportunities for improvement.

Introduction of Evidence-Based Management Philosophy

The personality and management philosophy of an organization are likely to reflect the personality of its executive leadership (Shortell and Kaluzny 2000). The new CEO subscribed enthusiastically to the potential contributions of disruptive innovation and had proven himself a successful turnaround-oriented leader in previous appointments. His two-month observation of St. Luke's revealed a generally complacent, underperforming enterprise, evidenced by quality and economic metrics out of the top decile or quartile of similar hospitals and health systems. In some instances, performance measures were considerably below the benchmarks required to move forward successfully.

At the special board meeting of August 2004 and a three-day board of directors retreat in January 2005, the CEO presented specific metrics associated with national performance benchmarks. The data used to compare St. Luke's performance included market share trends, operating margin trends, Joint Commission core measures, Press-Ganey scores, and total research expenditures.

The task list for management was substantial. The next 18 months were consumed by intramural struggles during which many managers and executives resisted the higher performance spotlight shining on many parts of the organization. They often resented the implied criticism of previous performance levels.

The CEO felt the hospital would improve once the new performance metrics were identified, agreed to, and embraced. He engaged several executive coaches to bring fresh eyes and enthusiasm to the process. He also assembled a team of executives, together with Baylor College of Medicine, and enrolled them in the action learning curriculum of the National Center for Healthcare Leadership organized at the University of Michigan's Ross School of Business by Professor Noel Tichy.

On March 28, 2005, the CEO spoke at a day-long conference of the health system's 200 department heads and executives. In what is described as his "Let a Thousand Flowers Bloom" speech, the CEO spent approximately 90 minutes working to motivate the full management team to critically assess historical performance, identify new paradigms for success, and press onward with the transformation necessary to ensure a vibrant future. The presentation centered on his belief that the organization would reach agreement on desired end points in collaboration with its board of directors. Most often, each area's management team would define the road traveled between current status and future objective. Managers would measure baseline performance and progress on the best available evidence.

As with any transformation of the scale envisioned, not all managers and executives present at the beginning of the critical journey would enter the promised land associated with top-performing hospitals. While it is beyond the scope of this chapter to provide a comprehensive review of the successes and failures experienced by St. Luke's and its leadership as the organization began its evolution, the sections that follow demonstrate how it used EB management as a transformational lever.

As noted by Rousseau, "evidence-based practice is a paradigm for making decisions that integrate the best available research evidence with decision maker expertise and client/customer preference to guide practice toward more desirable results" (Rousseau 2006). Unfortunately, he also notes, "evidence-based management can threaten managers' personal freedom to run their organizations as they see fit." In the authors' experience, EB management can be resisted precisely because it causes leaders to make decisions based on the best available scientific evidence rather than the individual's personal preference and experience. This is a Spockian illogic worthy of a Star Trek fantasy.

Evidence-Based Management in Action

EB management techniques were used in a number of different areas at St. Luke's, including the pharmacy, quality measurement, intensivist care, and formation of a comprehensive stroke program. Emphasis was given to identifying objective comparison data from a variety of sources.

Pharmacy

In 2004, a new director of pharmacy was recruited. The new director faced a special challenge, as the previous director of pharmacy was a favorite son of the organization and had been there nearly 20 years. As a large, tertiary (but fundamentally private-practice) hospital, St. Luke's did not have a history of strong formulary management. The hospital's leadership recognized financial opportunity in better management of its drug costs. They licensed a database from Solucient, a part of Thomson Healthcare, which analyzes operational data submitted by 800 healthcare organizations to show trends and make comparisons. This information promised to help the hospital establish appropriate benchmarks and identify where improvement was needed. With better metrics and a new director, the Pharmacy Department improved quickly.

In January 2005, the hospital installed an automated, unit-based cabinet system for medications throughout the hospital, which allowed 85 percent of frequently used medications to be stored on individual patient care units. Literature has shown that using these types of automated systems can improve safety, increase efficiency, reduce waste, and improve compliance with regulatory standards. Previously, many of these medications were sent from the pharmacy to the floor, which caused delays and missing doses, and in some cases affected quality of care. The new unit-based system reduced turnaround time for routine medications from 51 to 30 minutes and cut the previous year's number of missed doses by 70 percent.

The department sought ways to reduce drug costs through improved contract management. All General Purchasing Organization (GPO) commitments were reviewed to determine the greatest opportunities for savings and to ensure that formulary selection enabled achievement of market share requirements. Quarterly reviews with pharmaceutical manufacturers of high-dollar-usage drugs also gave the director the opportunity to negotiate savings beyond GPO contracts. Strict formulary management accompanied this effort, which required aligning physician prescribing with therapeutically equivalent contract products available.

The hospital reduced waste and benchmarked the results against historical organizational performance. For example, one project involved caspofungin, an anti-fungal drug administered intravenously. A process improvement team review revealed that caspofungin doses were frequently wasted. Often doses were scheduled to be administered in the late morning, when patients may have moved to a different bed or received discharge orders, and when nursing shifts typically change—all contributing to the potential for missed doses. By standardizing administration time of the drug to 6:00 a.m., the average waste per month decreased 57 percent, resulting in annual savings of $28,824. While not highly significant to the organizational bottom line, the project required no additional investment for implementation. These and other efforts resulted in pharmacy costs of $138.45 per adjusted patient day, $18 less than the Solucient comparison group average of $156.59. At the time, this figure ranked St. Luke's in the 29th percentile of the Solucient database comparison group.

The chief nursing officer reported long-standing concerns about the incidence of medication errors. The pharmacy director and her staff investigated which clinical areas presented the greatest opportunities for improvement and conducted a literature review to determine trends in medication errors. They knew that national measures indicated that approximately 13 percent of patients treated in the emergency department (ED) were admitted; at St. Luke's the rate was nearly 44 percent. This high rate of admission was reflected in the high case-mix index of patients at St. Luke's, which ranked in the 98th percentile in the Solucient database. The ED, therefore, presented an opportunity to streamline activities, not only to minimize medication errors but to optimize medication therapy.

In 2006, the American Society of Health-System Pharmacists published results from a national survey of hospital pharmacy departments that showed that 3.5 percent of hospitals directly allocated pharmacists to serve in the ED (Pedersen, Schneider, and Scheckelhoff 2006). This practice pays off: Ling and colleagues (2005) discovered that clinical interventions by ED pharmacists saved $579,000 per year, on average. This amount was based on the costs avoided by not having to treat adverse drug events. With this evidence, the director hypothesized that broadening clinical pharmacy services to the ED could positively influence both clinical and economic outcomes. Pharmacist interventions such as identification of contraindicated medications, as well as prevention of adverse drug reactions due to allergy, dosing errors, administering agent, and intolerance to medication, were identified as potential sources of savings.

Following the study, management recommended that St. Luke's add round-the-clock clinical and distributive pharmacy services in the ED. After the pilot period, the team concluded that adding a pharmacist and technician in the ED would result in a positive return on investment—avoiding an estimated $529,000 annually in costs—and improve quality of care. Leadership believed this figure to be a conservative estimate. During the first 10 days of the pilot alone, the pharmacy calculated a total cost avoidance of $37,641—an annualized savings of nearly $1.4 million, after adjusting for non-recurring first-year costs.

By focusing operations through the use of EB management interventions and benchmarking through the use of a performance dashboard of financial, clinical, and managerial measures, the Pharmacy Department decreased hospital-wide pharmaceutical costs per patient day to $134.72 in 2007, 3 percent less than in 2005, despite rising drug prices. St. Luke's remained in the 29th percentile (best one-third) of its Solucient comparison group, though meanwhile the Solucient comparison group average cost per patient day jumped to $163.15, a 4 percent increase from 2005. Though the organization is currently benchmarking against the 50th percentile, operational improvements will likely prompt leadership to narrow this target to the 25th percentile in the near future.

Quality Metrics

A full-time chief quality officer was hired at St. Luke's in 2006. This new position was designed to enhance evidence-based quality improvement efforts across the health system. An initial vision for quality improvement based on Donabedian's (1992) well-known structure-process-outcome methodology also was established.

Management created a three-year plan to develop infrastructure and improve quality and patient safety. The plan includes researching and analyzing evidence of quality improvement methods' effectiveness and assisting managers to implement those processes. One 2007 goal was to identify target populations for data collection. In addition to Centers for Medicare & Medicaid and Joint Commission core measures, data will be gathered on the spectrum of high-volume diagnosis-related groups at St. Luke's, including coronary artery bypass, percutaneous coronary intervention, cardiac catheterization lab procedures, automatic internal cardiac defibrillator, congestive heart failure, stroke, pulmonary, transplant, and orthopedics. Tracking these data will advance a quality-focused culture and provide an array of process and outcome indicators. With expanded metrics and such variety, management should be able to create an optimal strategy for quality measurement (Donabedian 1992). Furthermore, by performing these activities, St. Luke's will prepare for a potential shift from the current reimbursement system to the pay-for-performance approaches that reflect quality measures (Epstein, Lee, and Hamel 2004).

During the plan's second year, an inventory and benchmarking of procedures that define operations at St. Luke's will occur. As Chassin and Galvin (1998) stated in the Institute of Medicine (IOM) *National Roundtable Report*, "a notable constraint to quality improvement is posed by the lack of information infrastructure to support it in almost all healthcare delivery settings." Thus, developing an internal database to track quality, patient safety, and clinical and service excellence, and ensuring that all regulatory requirements and benchmarks are met, are key components in the second year.

By year three, St. Luke's will apply for the Malcolm Baldrige National Quality Award, given by the National Institute of Standards and Technology. This award recognizes organizations that excel in seven defined arenas: leadership; strategic planning; customer and market focus; measurement, analysis, and knowledge management; human resource focus; process management; and results. Although achievement of this award would be a considerable stretch in this time frame, the process is expected to create its own favorable Hawthorne effect within the main hospital.

ICU Intensivists

In response to rising healthcare costs and publications questioning the quality of U.S. healthcare, a group of corporations formed the Leapfrog Group in 2000 to use employer purchasing power as leverage on the healthcare industry to compel improvements in safety, quality, and customer value. Shortly thereafter, Leapfrog Hospital Insights were developed for five clinical areas—coronary artery bypass grafts, percutaneous coronary intervention, acute myocardial infarction, community-acquired pneumonia, and deliveries/newborn care—to assess quality, processes, and performance (Leapfrog Group 2006). With support from the Robert Wood Johnson Foundation and the Institute for Healthcare Improvement, Leapfrog has influenced consumer and purchaser choice and built a foundation for the potential shift to pay-for-performance.

One of the Insights tracked by Leapfrog has been performance on pneumonia-related quality measures, mostly based on Joint Commission core measures. One of the measures regards intensivist staffing in the intensive care unit (ICU). Evidence suggests that the use of such specialists in ICUs can improve mortality rates, length of stay, and hospital costs. Because of St. Luke's historically private practice orientation, attending physicians at St. Luke's have resisted the introduction of ICU intensivists. Although this resistance was initially viewed as a matter of financial territoriality, the hospital's outstanding outcome data prompted further examination of a potentially expensive addition to the cost infrastructure.

A review of the literature illustrates that many of the studies analyzing the intensivist model thus far have been limited in scope and have produced disease- or setting-specific outcomes. As suggested by Manthous (2004), Leapfrog's push for intensivists has been based more on "common sense and rational extrapolation of the data" as opposed to true scientific study and offers more of a "reasonable starting point for debate by physicians and policymakers about optimal methods of achieving intensivist-guided care of critically ill patients." Thus, despite its apparent success, the intensivist-led ICU model will need to be further evaluated before it gains enough evidence to become the standard of care.

St. Luke's has long employed an ICU staffing model that combines house staff with an experienced and aggressive nursing staff well-trained in pulmonary physiology. Approximately 25 percent of St. Luke's beds are in the ICU, which is a much higher proportion than at many other hospitals. For the last quarter of 2006, St. Luke's had a case-mix index of 1.84, ranking the hospital in the 98th percentile of patient acuity in the Solucient database. The organization has traditionally benchmarked against data from the Centers for Disease Control and Prevention (CDC), but is currently expanding to other databases, such as the University HealthSystem Consortium (UHC), to compare against similar facilities.

Notwithstanding Leapfrog's intensivist theory, St. Luke's ICUs have consistently performed better than benchmarks set by UHC without adopting such a model of care. In fact, its ICUs had lower-than-expected risk-adjusted mortality rates than the ICUs of all other healthcare organizations in the UHC Clinical Data Base in 2006. Leadership attributes this high level of performance to the ICUs' strong compliance with evidence-based pulmonary indicators and protocols developed over a decade ago by the hospital's respiratory therapy and infection control departments. These include ventilator bundling, spontaneous breathing trials, minimal sedation to reduce ventilator-acquired pneumonia (VAP), consistent prevention of pulmonary complications, and projects to reduce bloodstream infections. Evidence has shown that creating such a multifaceted approach to managing nosocomial infection plays a vital role in decreasing the overall spread of infection in endemic environments such as the ICU.

One of the key elements of these protocols is the "swish and swallow" process, in which all ICU patients are delivered an oral antiseptic to kill bacteria that lead to infection. After the administration of this protocol, follow-up surveillance cultures and chest X-rays are performed to discover any new infection. Most patients are found to have tracheobronchitis, a precursor to pneumonia, which early treatment can prevent. This system is a standard operating procedure in the ICUs. As a result of this protocol and others, healthcare-associated pneumonia rates fell from a high of 4 per 1,000 patient days to 0.05 per 1,000 patient days, and the rates were maintained for more than six years. VAP rates at St. Luke's, when benchmarked against similar healthcare facilities in CDC's database, consistently fall within the top 10 to 25 percent of hospitals. In this context, 24/7 intensivist staffing in St. Luke's ICUs at an annual base salary expense of $180,580 per physician must be questioned.

The system's chief quality officer expects to perform a study in conjunction with a university to analyze the processes and outcomes of one of St. Luke's ICUs and compare them, after risk adjustment, with ICU operations at another academic medical center that uses intensivists. This project should foster a growing evidence base to better understand intensivist versus non-intensivist models in academic health settings and test the hypothesis that it is possible to go against the grain yet still achieve high performance.

Building a Comprehensive Stroke Program

Cardiac services have been the historical flagship services of St. Luke's, but other product lines eventually were needed to grow and stabilize the organization, both financially and operationally. One area that senior leadership identified was neurological services.

In the past decade, the Joint Commission has instituted several disease-specific certification programs, incorporating goals discussed in the literature about enhancing benefits to patients by standardizing treatments. To accomplish such consistency, the Joint Commission created the Certificate of Distinction for Primary Stroke Centers to award organizations that met defined benchmarks and performance measures related to processes and outcomes.

In general, the literature supports the use of disease-specific quality measurement. The IOM (2001) *Crossing the Quality Chasm* report predicts that focus on improving the quality of care for specific common conditions is most likely to produce the greatest results. A review of more recent literature also suggests that creating a "coordinated hospital-based program or system is likely to improve outcomes of patients with strokes and complex cerebrovascular disease" (Alberts et al. 2005). Senior management at St. Luke's saw a critical opportunity to become an early adopter of this approach—to grow a small but promising practice that already existed at the hospital into a comprehensive stroke center.

Stroke program managers worked in conjunction with senior leadership, physicians, and other clinical staff to gain buy-in for the comprehensive stroke center vision. There was some resistance from those who wanted to remain a small program, but physician champions helped shift the culture. Eventually, leadership decided that working toward the common goal of improving patient care was not only important, but vital for the future sustainability of operations. Thus, tracking the necessary Joint Commission benchmarks, which were based on evidence reported by the American Stroke Association and the Brain Attack Coalition, became a key task of neurological units, as a prerequisite for applying for the new Joint Commission certification.

To apply for Joint Commission certification, organizations were required to measure performance in 12 areas and achieve 80 percent compliance in all 12 over a four-month period. Managers of the stroke program also used benchmarking data from the Advisory Board Company and other widely accepted sources to create a broad base of evidence that could be used to improve the program. The evidence led to the development of a set of best practices for standardizing patient care.

St. Luke's achieved the necessary compliance rates to apply for certification and in 2004 became one of two Houston-area hospitals to earn a certificate of distinction for primary stroke centers after an exhaustive Joint Commission on-site review. In October 2007, the program earned a five-star rating from HealthGrades, in addition to ranking number one in the state of Texas out of 213 ranked facilities. Treatment at St. Luke's now includes neuroradiological interventions, and there is new support for building a neurosciences center based on the stroke program's fundamentals.

Facility Design

U.S. hospital construction expenditures are projected to exceed $20 billion per year over the next decade, necessitating a shift from design guesswork to *evidence-based design*, a concept in which architects, planners, and interior designers base their decisions on research that links aspects of the physical environment to positive patient, staff, and community measures. In 2005, St. Luke's joined the Center for Health Design's (CHD) Pebble Project. Member organizations perform studies and document research findings to inform designers, administrators, researchers, and facility managers about successful facility design strategies. With more than 40 members as of August 2007, CHD (2006) believes a nexus of communication and dialog regarding building design will facilitate developing a body of evidence for organizations to use in the design of healthcare facilities. As a "Pebble," St. Luke's has access to the wealth of information on organizational transformation, clinical advances, financial measures, and satisfaction of employees and patients. Findings indicate that well-researched design can enhance patient experience and improve employee productivity and operational and financial performance.

St. Luke's Architecture and Construction Services Department (ACSD) has been involved in developing plans since 2001 to build the new Patient Care Center (PCC) on the Texas Medical Center campus. This project will require demolition of the original hospital structure, known as the "1954 Building." In designing the PCC, ACSD's goal is to create a facility that best meets the needs of patients and staff according to available evidence, within the confines of land and budget constraints.

The team has been through several plan iterations since 2005. In particular, ACSD has paid close attention to the evidence analyzing clinical outcomes associated with private versus non-private rooms. Evaluation of findings in more than 120 studies has revealed convincing evidence that single-bed rooms lower nosocomial infection rates, in part because they are easier to decontaminate and cross-contamination between room occupants is reduced.

Sound control has been another key issue addressed by the ACSD group. Its goal is to create an environment in which sound control protects patient privacy and confidentiality and minimizes noise from alarms, pagers, and activities on the unit, since "high noise levels negatively impact patient and staff health and well-being and may slow the process of healing among patients" (Joseph and Ulrich 2007). Sound-control strategies include construction of private rooms to enhance confidentiality, integration of noise-absorbing materials into construction, training employees to be conscious of noise levels, and installation of floor-to-ceiling walls to minimize sound travel. ACSD staff is attempting to use this evidence as a cornerstone in the development of plans for the Patient Care Center and other upcoming projects.

St. Luke's has had experience with evidence-based design theories. The plans for a 100-bed St. Luke's Sugar Land Hospital are one example. All patient rooms in the facility will be same-handed, which means each will have exactly the same layout, in contrast to prevailing trends for mirror-image rooms in which bathrooms are back-to-back and patient's headwalls are common to one another (which means that the layout of gas lines and other headwall functions is reversed from one room to the next). Another concern is how room design and appointments can reduce patient falls, more than 40 percent of which occur as patients move or are transferred to and from the bed. While there is no definitive evidence supporting same-handed rooms in the healthcare literature, due to space issues at the Sugar Land site, this design yielded the shortest bed-to-toilet distance in every room. More evidence will be necessary to evaluate and establish the cost benefit of the incremental investment.

The universal room concept, which enables treatment of easy to complex patients in any room (eliminating the need for multiple transfers to intensive care and step-down units), has been a source of frustration at St. Luke's. During the initial planning phase of the Patient Care Center, ACSD proposed to implement a universal room design. This layout would create flexibility, enable closure of units during future construction, and accommodate changes in long-term census or patient population. However, due to lack of evidence-based support for the concept, its high associated costs, and its high space demands, this approach was abandoned.

Although costs and limited space remain important considerations for St. Luke's, using evidence promoted by Pebble Project research and others has allowed the organization to initiate a more patient-focused approach to building design.

Employee Engagement

St. Luke's partnered with the Gallup Organization in 2001 to track employee engagement. From 2004 to 2006, Gallup surveyed more than 5 million employees in 455 organizations around the world, using the "Q12," a standard, web-based survey of 12 questions designed through 30 years of quantitative and qualitative research to correlate to turnover and retention, customer metrics, safety, productivity, and profitability. Annually, Gallup calculates a "grand mean" using data from all of the organizations in its national healthcare database to create employee engagement benchmarks for comparison among organizations. Gallup research has produced evidence that organizations with greater employee engagement have lower patient mortality and complication indexes, fewer nosocomial infections, improved patient satisfaction, and better financial performance. Additionally, healthcare organizations with greater employee engagement have 10 to 26 percent less turnover, grow profit from 8 to 15 percent, and increase productivity from 6 to 11 percent. Furthermore, the survey predicts patient mortality rates on the basis of nurses' engagement level, the number of nurses per patient day, and the percentage of overtime hours per year.

After the first round of the survey in 2001, St. Luke's human resources (HR) department divided employees into work groups based on area of employment. The employees took the survey, and administrators used the results to create a plan for improvement based on one strength and one weakness the survey revealed. An online tool allowed managers to select one of the 12 questions, and then delivered a set of researched, best-practice guidelines for achieving improvement in that question's performance area. Managers also used the tool to develop an action timeline and were encouraged to enter dates of completion for specific tasks to ensure adherence to the schedule.

In 2007, 86 percent of St. Luke's 4,800 employees participated. Although opportunities for improvement have been identified using a number of Gallup metrics, St. Luke's employee engagement ratio (3.15:1, engaged:unengaged) slightly outpaced other organizations in the Gallup health data set (average, 3:1) and the U.S. working population (average, 2:1). Interestingly, the engagement ratio for St. Luke's nurses (3.64:1) is higher than for the average U.S. RNs (1.94:1) and for nurses in the Gallup healthcare database (3:1).

In total, the percentage of engaged employees at St. Luke's increased by 3 percent between 2005 and 2007. Still, only 28 percent of employees reported total satisfaction, below the 43 percent benchmark that represents the 75th percentile of the healthcare data group. However, this figure is consistent with Gallup's overall findings for the healthcare industry, which has experienced declining overall satisfaction but improving employee engagement since 1999. Gallup findings for St. Luke's also showed that grand mean scores for executives and managers were higher than for supervisors and lower-level employees. To improve the overall engagement score, Gallup recommended a focus on efforts to engage their direct reports through one-on-one development and goal setting based on clear expectations of performance and accountability.

Achieving such a high level of overall participation gives St. Luke's leadership a strong start on creating strategies for the development of human capital within the organization. Additionally, St. Luke's is moving forward with plans to become a study site for Gallup, which will allow for in-depth research into site-specific aspects of employee engagement.

Nurse Placement

Since 1998, the United States has been in the midst of a growing nursing shortage. The federal government predicts that the country will have a million fewer nurses than needed by 2020. The American Hospital Association recently reported a national RN vacancy rate of 8.5 percent (American Hopital Association 2006). In 2006, a Texas Department of State Health Services survey found a statewide RN turnover rate of 18.2 percent for the 226 reporting hospitals, up from 15.6 percent in 2004 (Texas Center for Nursing Workforce Studies 2008.) The importance of mitigating the effects of these trends cannot be overstated.

As noted by Needleman and colleagues (2002), "a higher proportion of hours of nursing care provided by registered nurses and a greater number of hours of care by registered nurses per day are associated with better care for hospitalized patients." Another study correlated lower mortality rates with staffing at a 4:1 (patient:nurse) ratio as opposed to 6:1, with an expected "2.3 additional deaths per 1,000 patients and 8.7 additional deaths per 1,000 patients with complications" when nurses must care for more patients (Aiken et al. 2002). Additionally, the costs of improving staffing ratios may be at least partially offset by reduced costs associated with turnover and recruitment—estimated anywhere from $40,000 to $64,000 per nurse, depending on skill level.

Like most hospitals, St. Luke's has felt pressures associated with these shortages. In 2003, the hospital's RN turnover rate was 12.5 percent, near the higher end of estimates at the time. St. Luke's instituted a specialized HR function directed at nursing recruitment and retention, staffed by several RNs. After researching various hiring practices, the HR team decided to focus on critical needs of applicants through a program called Organization Fit. Evidence has shown that staff members' acclimation to their team, job, and organization strongly affects work attitudes (Kovner 2001). When needs are met at these levels, more employees will have a constructive experience and become engaged in their work.

In 2003, St. Luke's partnered with the Center for Talent Retention, which developed a set of 50 "critical needs" based on four areas. These categories included work aspects, manager relations, employee needs, and the organization. The HR team convened a focus group with nursing staff of each nursing unit, excluding managers, to determine which of the critical needs were best being met. After compiling these data, HR administered the critical needs survey to potential nursing hires. Candidates were asked to rate their top ten critical needs. From these ratings, HR matched the candidate with the unit that would best meet those needs.

The first year after the Organization Fit process for nursing hires was instituted, nursing attrition declined from 12.5 to 9.6 percent. Though additional HR efforts to redesign hiring practices also affected retention, Organization Fit likely played a role. Similarly, the Gallup survey indicates that the level of nurses' engagement has increased steadily since the implementation of Organization Fit. Moving forward, metrics related to nursing turnover, recruitment, and retention will be followed closely to determine long-term trends and whether the evidence supports using Organization Fit as a best practice at St. Luke's.

Summary

In this chapter, we noted how the adoption of EB management forms a "state religion" in which employees, managers, and executives are encouraged to use the literature available to them to better inform decision making.

St. Luke's projects show how a complex health system moves toward EB management. In the pharmacy, national data permit comparison of drug cost per patient day and facilitate evaluation of professional staffing alternatives in the ED and their impact on cost and quality. In the formation of a new quality assurance program, the literature provides templates for program design and best practices.

In the ICUs, St. Luke's data are used to step back from a Leapfrog-inspired intensivist staffing goal because other less costly institutional practices are achieving favorable outcomes. In three years, a stroke program has been developed from the ground up, first achieving 80 percent compliance with a series of Joint Commission national criteria and subsequently realizing first position among 213 ranked programs in Texas. A growing and publicly recognized reputation for high quality has contributed to a 47 percent volume increase in stroke care.

A $250 million facilities investment at St. Luke's Episcopal Hospital and a $100 million investment in the new St. Luke's Sugar Land Hospital have been informed by the findings of the national Pebble Project, with respect to how certain design considerations improve quality of care, employee well-being, and patient and staff satisfaction. St. Luke's will be an active and continuing contributor to the evolving literature on the subject.

The engagement of St. Luke's employees has been measured against a large set of comparison organizations. The results, containing a mix of good and bad news for the hospital, demonstrate strengths, weaknesses, opportunities, and threats. Goals and objectives for improvement are based on this evidence, and progress will be measured each year.

Finally, new nurses are placed on patient units that best match their needs, which has contributed to reductions in turnover and associated costs. Although evidence in the development of screening and assignment tools has been well used, St. Luke's needs to measure turnover statistics and weighting of contributing factors.

Conclusion

Archimedes is attributed with first understanding that one could move the world given an appropriate lever and fulcrum. In a considerably more modest context, many senior healthcare executives at some point in a 30- to 40-year professional career will find themselves in business circumstances requiring major organizational transformation. These fixes may be "rescues" of failing enterprises or "renovations" of underperforming institutions.

Increasing numbers of specialty consulting firms and practitioners make careers of such management situations. All healthcare executives seeking to identify and apply transformational leverage must motivate employees and managers to achieve the improved performance levels needed for organizational sustainability. The goal is not merely to survive, but to thrive. Organizations must not only have healthy financial statements, but also deliver the high-quality care required by external accreditation organizations. The growing demand for accountability set forth by such external entities further necessitates the use of EB management.

The most critical dimension to organizational transformation is recognition and acceptance of a problem. EB management provides the fulcrum on which improvement can be leveraged. Information sources to support healthcare organizations in this quest are increasingly abundant. Among them are useful metrics reported or developed by industry affinity groups such as the University HealthSystem Consortium and the American Society of Health-System Pharmacists. Commercial products are available from an increasing number of consulting and data engineering firms. Government databases can be expected to assume a more influential position, although most publicly reported data have limitations derived from residual nonstandard or unverified data classification processes. As these impediments to programmatic comparison are progressively resolved, EB management will become an ever more useful tool.

References

Aiken, L. H., S. P. Clarke, D. M. Sloane, J. Sochalski, and J. H. Silber. 2002. "Hospital Nurse Staffing and Patient Mortality, Nurse Burnout, and Job Dissatisfaction." *Journal of the American Medical Association* 288 (16): 1987–93.

Alberts, M. A., R. E. Latchaw, W. R. Selman, T. Shephard, M. N. Hadley, L. M. Brass, W. Koroshetz, J. R. Marler, J. Booss., R. D. Zorowitz, J. B. Croft, E. Magnis, D. Mulligan, A. Jagoda, R. O'Connor, C. M. Cawley, J. J. Connors, J. A. Rose-DeRenzy, M. Emr, M. Warren, and M. D. Walker. 2005. "Recommendations for Comprehensive Stroke Centers: A Consensus Statement from the Brain Attack Coalition." *Stroke* 36: 1597–1618.

Center for Health Design (CHD). 2006. "The Pebble Project®." [Online information; retrieved 08/07/07.] www.healthdesign.org/research/pebble/partners.php.

Chassin, M. R., and R. W. Galvin. 1998. "The Urgent Need to Improve Healthcare Quality: Institute of Medicine National Roundtable on Healthcare Quality." *Journal of the American Medical Association* 280 (11): 1000–05.

Donabedian, A. 1992. "The Role of Outcomes in Quality Assessment and Assurance." *Quality Review Board* 11: 356–60.

Epstein, A. M., T. H. Lee, and M. B. Hamel. 2004. "Paying Physicians for High-Quality Care." *New England Journal of Medicine* 350 (4): 406–10

Institute of Medicine (IOM). 2001. *Crossing the Quality Chasm: A New Health System for the 21st Century.* Washington, DC: National Academies Press.

Joseph, A., and R. Ulrich. 2007. "Sound Control for Improved Outcomes in Healthcare Settings." The Center for Health Design. Issue Paper 14.

Kovner, C. 2001. "The Impact of Staffing and the Organization of Work on Patient Outcomes and Healthcare Workers in Healthcare Organizations." *The Joint Commission Journal on Quality Improvement* 27: 458–68.

Leapfrog Group. 2006. "Leapfrog Hospital Insights Fact Sheet." [Online article or information; retrieved 08/14/07.] https://leapfrog.medstat .com/insights/references/FactSheet.doc.

Ling, J. M., L. A. Mike, J. Rubin, P. Abraham, A. Howe, J. Patka, and D. Vigliotti. 2005. "Documentation of Pharmacist Interventions in the Emergency Department." *American Journal of Health-System Pharmacy* 62 (17): 1793-97.

Manthous, C. 2004. "Leapfrog and Critical Care: Evidence- and Reality-Based Intensive Care for the 21st Century." *American Journal of Medicine* 116: 188–93.

Needleman, J., P. Buerhaus, S. Mattke, M. Stewart, and K. Zelevinsky. 2002. "Nurse-Staffing Levels and the Quality of Care in Hospitals." *New England Journal of Medicine* 346 (22): 1715–22.

Pedersen, C. A., P. H. Schneider, and D. J. Scheckelhoff. 2006. "ASHP National Survey of Pharmacy Practice in Hospital Settings: Dispensing and Administration—2005." *American Journal of Health-System Pharmacy* 63: 327–45.

Rousseau, D. M. 2006. "Is There Such a Thing as Evidence-Based Management?" *Academy of Management Review* 31 (2): 258.

Shortell, S. M., and A. D. Kaluzny. 2000. *Healthcare Management: Organization Design and Behavior*, 4th edition. Albany, NY: Delmar.

EVIDENCE-BASED MANAGEMENT AT TWO NEW YORK CITY MEDICAL CENTERS

Anthony R. Kovner

Introduction

For 16 years, I've served as a management consultant to Montefiore Medical Center in the Bronx and as a board member of another hospital in Brooklyn, New York. At the second hospital, I have been a member of the Executive Committee, chairman of the Performance Improvement Committee, and vice chairman of the HMO Committee. Although I lack detailed knowledge about precisely how decision making works at these two institutions "on the inside," I have observed over time the two hospitals' very different approaches to decision making. Consider my observations the 20,000-foot view.

Neither Montefiore nor the other hospital has a strategy to implement evidence-based management (EB management). No individual manager is responsible for EB management. There is no accountability process for EB management. When administrators consider major management interventions, they do not follow the six-step EB management process. Nevertheless, managers at both systems have told me they use EB management, even if they don't use the same terminology or follow the typical step-wise progression. According to the Davenport/Harris "competing on analytic stages model," I would rank both organizations as being at Stage 2—that is, organizations that use localized analytics that may or may not be supporting the hospital's distinctive capabilities (Davenport and Harris 2007; see charts, pp. 36, 114).

Montefiore Medical Center

To better understand the decision-making process used at Montefiore, I interviewed Steve Safyer, the hospital's chief medical officer. To his information, I added my own insights from my long-standing consultancy with this organization.

According to Dr. Safyer, a version of EB management is practiced at Montefiore. "I am an intuitive thinker," he says. "Intuitive thinking has a valuable contribution to make, but I could stray, if left to my own." He says decision making is conducted by teams "made up of people with different skill sets and approaches to problems and leadership." Team members range from accountants and finance types to clinical staff—doctors and nurses. The top management team includes six or seven individuals—all top executives of their respective departments: legal, finance, operations, medicine, and the chief executive. This structure has been in place for the past several years.

As Dr. Safyer describes the decision process, "Our President 'plants the flag,' indicating where we are going to stand on important strategic issues. Then we plan and implement our strategy. Take, for example, the decision to acquire another hospital. We go through every one of the EB management steps." At Montefiore, the Executive Committee wrestles long and hard with such key decisions. "We're plan-driven and rigorous in our large discussions. We're all equal in the discussion and free to express ourselves. Once a strategic decision has been made, we unite around the hospital's approach to an issue." The executive team may vote on this, but Dr. Safyer says the president has 51 percent of the vote.

Here are some of the sentinel decisions Montefiore has made over the last 15 years, for which Dr. Safyer reports an evidence-based approach was used:

- The development of a large primary care network (Analysis revealed the hospital would lose money on the project, but it correctly predicted those losses would be offset by additional admissions.)
- A decision to accept 100,000 patients from a local HMO—one-third of whom would have to change their site of care—which required a thorough risk analysis and feasibility assessment
- Migration to a digital information system to improve quality, safety, and good business practices
- A decision to move toward an integrated delivery system
- Withdrawal from large contracts to provide medical services for the New York City Health and Hospitals Corporation (a public hospital system) and for the prisoner health facility on Riker's Island
- Decisions in 1993 and thereafter not to merge or acquire another hospital, which was the prevailing trend in New York City at that time, despite the financial benefit and risk protection a merger or an acquisition would have provided
- The decision more than a decade later to acquire Our Lady of Mercy Hospital, under circumstances different from those of the early 1990s

Regarding the decision to acquire Our Lady of Mercy, Dr. Safyer explained that, by 2005, Montefiore increased the volume of inpatient admissions and decreased lengths of stay. The hospital business is one of high fixed costs. Because costs are rising faster than revenues, hospitals have to increase the volume of services it provides. The hospital was functioning at 100 percent capacity and, compared to its competitors, had the shortest length of stay. For example, two area competitors—each with approximately the same number of beds as Montefiore (about 1,000)—discharged 45,000–50,000 patients per year, whereas Montefiore discharged more than 65,000. "We had hit a wall financially and couldn't grow the business under our financial model without expanding capacity," he said.

Dr. Safyer described the decision-making process top management followed in considering the merger with Our Lady of Mercy, using the template of EB management:

1. Framing the question behind the decision

It was clear to the management team that the basic question was "how much would it cost to acquire 200 to 300 additional beds?" Building a new facility was impossible, given the difficulties in acquiring land and obtaining a certificate of need from the state, at a time when a governor's commission was recommending the closure of hospital beds.

2. Finding sources of information

"We did extensive due diligence," Dr. Safyer said. "We looked into every aspect of Our Lady of Mercy. We investigated community issues, where the patients came from and the kinds of illnesses they had, what kinds of referrals we could expect, who served on the hospital's medical staff, where they practiced and whether they had existing relationships with Montefiore, the condition of the hospital's plant and facilities, its management structure." By the end of the process, he said, "We felt we knew more than their own management and board had ever known about how the institution had been functioning!"

3. Assessing the accuracy of the information

Because Montefiore had just built its own children's hospital, management believed it had solid, current information about the climate for raising money, obtaining state approvals, and financing a new building. Still, Dr. Safyer said, "We met with focus groups and with all their hospital's external stake-holders. These included the debt people, the accountants and consultants, the lending agencies, the banks, the Federal Housing Administration, the state health department. We met extensively with some of the leaders on their board." Top management was willing to take the time to verify the information they had collected, in part because they were not in a crisis situation. "We had enough slack in our regular management positions and capable subordinates to devote to validating this information."

4. Assessing the applicability and actionability of the information

The potential merger partner was located in the Bronx, Montefiore's familiar home borough. In the past it had merged with another hospital, had run medical services under contract with the City of New York at two other hospitals, and had set up a primary care network. Management recognized that geographic propinquity would have to be an essential part of the deal and therefore did not consider organizations from other geographic areas.

Three major stakeholders would make or break the deal, Dr. Safyer said: Montefiore's management and board; the Catholic archdiocese, which owned Our Lady of Mercy; and the state's governor. The archdiocese would have to deal with the unwanted problems of a failing hospital. It didn't want the hospital to go bankrupt, nor did it want to abandon Catholic principles of care. The hospital also wanted to continue with its mission, and the state health department recognized that the part of the Bronx it served sorely needed hospital services. The governor was running for president, and the archdiocese's goodwill was important.

With all these forces in play, an agreement was reached whereby Montefiore helped the hospital avoid bankruptcy, the archdiocese relinquished financial liability, the governor achieved a solution that the archdiocese favored, and the state health department helped cover operating losses during a transition period.

5. Determining whether top management has adequate information

On the basis of the foregoing, Montefiore management believed it knew enough to begin the merger process. Because that process is still under way, Montefiore must wait before it can move on to step 6, evaluating the results.[1]

I concluded the interview by asking Dr. Safyer how EB management techniques fit into Montefiore's future. He said, "We can always improve what we are doing, but we have a good formula for framing and deciding strategic issues and a solid and experienced management team." Montefiore continues to face challenges that EB management could address, including capacity problems, malpractice costs, low Medicaid reimbursements, the need to provide community health services, the desire to build a closer relationship with Albert Einstein College of Medicine, and the need to expand some specialty services, like organ transplants. "We need to build out excellence," he concluded.

The Other Hospital

The second hospital in this comparison has $1.5 billion in annual revenues. The health center is located in southwest Brooklyn. Its main components are a 425-bed hospital, a 200-bed nursing home, a large federally funded and closely affiliated (but not owned) neighborhood health center, and a Medicaid HMO with more than 250,000 members.

According to its 2006 annual report, the hospital is "committed to providing high-quality, culturally competent healthcare and support services to the communities of southwest Brooklyn." It is reasonably well managed, certainly as far as New York City hospitals go. Many of my former students work as managers there, and I was heavily involved on the search committee that five years ago recruited the current CEO. However, the hospital has not applied EB management well. One key example concerns the potential sale of its HMO.

In 2003, the hospital was considering selling its HMO, simply because the hospital needed money. The HMO had been contributing up to $10 million per year to the hospital's bottom line, but this number was decreasing significantly for a variety of reasons. The hospital needed money because of operating losses caused in part by several poor decisions by the board and previous administration. The problems were exacerbated by rising malpractice premiums (the hospital was self-insured) and pension fund contributions (the fund was inadequately subsidized).

The hospital's top management recommended selling the HMO because at that time, investor-owned companies were purchasing Medicaid HMOs in other locations for relatively large amounts. The board agreed to put the HMO on the market at a price of $300 million, but might have accepted considerably less. Three years later, after hundreds of hours of board discussions with various sets of consultants, bankers, and lawyers, the HMO failed to sell.

Board members who opposed the sale were accused of "not being part of the team." These board members were dissatisfied with the health system's financial performance over several years and its lack of investment in the HMO, which might have contributed to poor operating results. The opponents also wanted the sale proceeds to go toward building a new hospital to replace the current obsolete facility, rather than reversing existing deficits.

Board leadership and top management apparently gave little thought to several key issues: (1) what the hospital would do with the proceeds if the HMO were sold, (2) other alternatives to solve the health system's financial problems, such as sale or divestiture of the hospital, and (3) how the substantial contributions of HMO surpluses to hospital operations could have been invested (or would be invested in the future) to expand the HMO's markets or improve its products.

By not following the step-wise EB management process, which ensures that managers and boards have accurate and adequate information for decision making, the hospital was unable to come to grips with the issues around the proposed sale—at an enormous cost in time and effort for everyone involved, not to mention steep opportunity costs.

Conclusion

This comparison between Montefiore and the other New York City hospital reveals the value of EB management, even when it is applied selectively. Montefiore is stronger and more financially stable because of its careful use of EB management. The other hospital, while generally well managed, could be more successful if it applied EB management in certain situations.

End Note

1. Our Lady of Mercy had debts of $70 to $80 million. Montefiore could not invest in it because Montefiore could not be repaid if Our Lady of Mercy went bankrupt.

Reference

Davenport, T., and J. G. Harris. 2007. *Competing on Analytics*. Boston: Harvard Business School Press.

THEORIES AND DEFINITIONS OF EVIDENCE-BASED MANAGEMENT

EVIDENCE-BASED MANAGEMENT RECONSIDERED

Anthony R. Kovner and Thomas G. Rundall

This chapter is a reprint of an article from the Spring 2006 issue of Frontiers of Health Services Management. *Reprinted with permission.*

SUMMARY. Reports of medical mistakes have splashed across newspapers and magazines in the United States. At the same time, instances of overuse, underuse, and misuse of management tactics and strategies receive far less attention. The sense of urgency associated with improving the quality of medical care does not exist with respect to improving the quality of management decision making. A more evidence-based approach would improve the competence of the decision-makers and their motivation to use more scientific methods when making a decision. The authors of this article consider a study of 68 U.S. health services managers that found a low level of evidence-based management behaviors. From the findings, four strategies are suggested to increase health systems managers' use of research evidence to improve decision making: focusing evidence-based decision making on strategically important issues, developing committees and other structures to diffuse management research throughout the organization, building a management culture that values research, and training managers in the competencies required to apply research evidence to health services management decisions. To aid the manager in understanding and applying an evidence-based approach to decision making, the article provides practical tools, techniques, and resources for immediate use.

What we do for and with patients and how we organize those efforts should, to the extent possible, be based on knowledge of what works. Put differently, both the application of clinical medicine and the application of organizational behavior should be evidence based.

> Stephen M. Shortell, Ph.D., FACHE (Shortell 2001)

What discourages our use of research is something that is typical of all health systems. That is, we are on a rapid cycle...We don't have two years to study something. Sometimes having 40 percent of the information on something may be enough. We make a decision and change it if it doesn't work.

> Health system manager (Kovner 2005)

The numerous developments in evidence-based decision making over the past decade should influence health organization leaders and managers to explicitly incorporate such decision making in their management processes. For example, the considerable use of evidence-based decision making by physicians has resulted in the proliferation of patient care guidelines and related decision-support materials for physicians (Sackett et al. 1996; Friedland et al. 1998; Sackett et al. 2000; Geyman, Deyo, and Ramsey 2000; Eddy 2005; AHRQ 2006a). Acceptance of the evidence-based approach has been growing in nursing, public health, health policy making, and other specialty areas in the health sciences (Lomas 2000; Donaldson, Mugford, and Vale 2002; Lavis et al. 2002; Stewart 2002; Lavis et al. 2003; Brownson et al. 2003; Muir Gray 2004; Shojania and Grimshaw 2005; Hatcher and Oakley-Browne 2005; Fox 2005). As Muir Gray suggests (2004), an evidence-based approach would improve the competence of decision-makers and their motivation to use more scientific methods when making a decision. In their recent book, *Management Mistakes in Healthcare*, Paul Hofmann and Frankie Perry call for the identification, correction, and prevention of management mistakes in healthcare (Hofmann and Perry 2005). Moreover, articles have appeared in health management and health services research journals urging health services managers to examine the nature of decision making in their organizations and to consider adopting an evidence-based approach (Axelson 1998; Davies and Nutley 1999; Kovner, Elton, and Billings 2000; Walshe and Rundall 2001; Greenhalgh et al. 2004; Muir Gray 2004; Clancy and Cronin 2005). Web-based sources of evidence for managers have emerged, including compendiums of primary research studies and research syntheses developed by the Agency for Healthcare Research and Quality (AHRQ) (www.ahrq.gov/research), the Cochrane Effective Practice and Organization of Care Group (www.epoc.uottawa.ca), and others. Federal agencies have supported research to improve quality, safety, and efficiency in the organization and delivery of health services (AHRQ 2006b). For example, since 2000 AHRQ has funded the Integrated Delivery System Research Network (IDSRN), now "Accelerating Change and Transformation in Organizations and Networks" (ACTION), which was explicitly designed to create, support, and disseminate scientific evidence about what works and what does not work. Since 1991 the Center for Health Management Research (depts.washington.edu/chmr/about), a National Science Foundation–funded Industry-University Research Collaborative, has been facilitating collaborative research among university-based health services researchers and health system managers. Finally, evidence-based decision making has been increasingly incorporated into lists of competencies necessary for effective management of modern health services organizations. The management competencies proposed by the Healthcare Leadership Alliance (2005) include acquiring, appraising, and applying research findings to management decisions.[1] Similarly, the Health Leadership Competency Model, developed by the National Center for Healthcare Leadership (2004), incorporates competencies supporting evidence-based decision making, most notably the competency referred to as "analytical thinking":

> The ability to understand a situation, issue, or problem by breaking it into smaller pieces or tracing its implications in a step-by-step way. It includes organizing the parts of a situation, issues, or problem systematically; making systematic comparisons of different features or aspects; setting priorities on a rational basis; and identifying time sequences, causal relationships, or if-then relationships.

Similar developments are unfolding in the health systems of other developed countries. Indeed, if anything, countries with national health insurance and/or a public delivery system have developed more resources than the United States for evidence-based healthcare management. For example, the United Kingdom National Health Service has established the NHS Service Delivery and Organization Programme (www.sdo.lshtm.ac.uk), the U.K. National Library for Health (www.nelh.nhs.uk), and the Health Management Online resource within the National Health Service in Scotland (www.healthmanagementonline.co.uk), and the Canadian government has established the Canadian Health Services Research Foundation (www.chsrf.ca).

Recent research in the United Kingdom and in Canada suggests that health managers and policy makers make little use of the evidence-based approach to decision making and, indeed, reveals a wide gap between the health services research and health policy and management communities (Lavis, et al. 2002; Canadian Health Services Research Foundation 2000; 2004). In those countries, a number of steps have been identified that could increase the uptake of evidence-based healthcare management. For example, the Canadian Health Services Research Foundation (2000, 7) suggests:

> [D]ecision makers need to find more effective ways to organize and communicate their priorities and problems, while researchers and research funders must develop mechanisms to access information on these priorities and problems and turn them into research activity. …Researchers need to learn how to simplify their findings and demonstrate their application to the health system in order to communicate better with decision makers and knowledge purveyors. …The knowledge purveyors have to improve their ability to screen and appraise information—to sort the facts from the stories. …Decision makers and their organizations need to improve their capacity to receive such appraised and screened information and to act upon it.

Moreover, studies in Canada and the United Kingdom have noted the substantial differences between health services managers and health services researchers in their understandings of what is considered evidence, what type of systematic review of evidence is helpful to decision makers, and the extent to which management and policy decision making can and should be evidence based (Canadian Health Services Research Foundation 2005; Sheldon 2005; Mays, Pope, and Popay 2005; Pawson et al. 2005; Lavis et al. 2005).

No study of U.S. health services managers' perspectives on evidence-based decision making exists, hence, we have little evidence to guide us in developing strategies to strengthen understanding and use of EB management among health services managers. The purposes of this article are four-fold: (1) to briefly describe the EB management approach; (2) to describe the questions to which EB management can be applied; (3) to report on a recent study conducted by one of the authors (Kovner 2005) to understand better the use of evidence in decision making by health services managers; and (4) to suggest a number of practical strategies that U.S. health services organizations can use to implement or strengthen an evidence-based approach to decision making in their organization.

What Is Evidence-Based Management?

Evidence-based management applies the idea of evidence-based decision making to business process, operational, and strategic decisions in health services organizations. Simply put, EB management is the systematic application of the best available evidence to the evaluation of managerial strategies for improving the performance of health services organizations. What distinguishes EB management from other approaches to decision making is the notion that whenever possible, health services managers should incorporate into their decision making evidence from well-conducted management research. It must be emphasized that other sources of information and knowledge, such as personal experience, experiences of others in similar situations, expert opinion, and simple inspection of data trends and patterns, can and should be used if such information is the best available evidence for a given decision. As is the case with evidence-based medicine, the research evidence one uses in EB management does not replace but rather complements other types of knowledge and information.

The EB management approach recognizes that decision making is a process rather than a simple act of choosing among alternatives. Under ideal circumstances, this process involves a number of steps. Figures 5.1 and 5.2 depict the contribution of the EB management approach to two frequently used decision-making processes in health organizations.

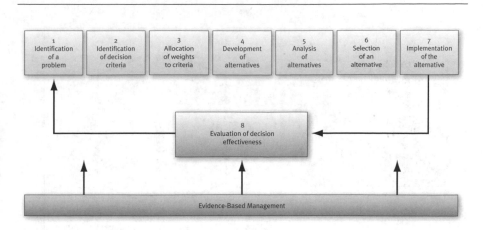

FIGURE 5.1
The Eight Step
Decision-
Making Process

SOURCE: Adapted from Robbins and DeCenzo (2004, 106).

The decision-making process begins with the identification of a problem (step 1), or more specifically, identification of the discrepancy between an existing and a desired state of affairs. The decision maker(s) uses various techniques, types of information, analyses, and actions to complete the cycle, with information gained from an evaluation of the decision (step 8) helping to determine whether the problem continues to exist in the future. Of special interest to the field of EB management are steps 5 and 6. The promise of EB management is that by incorporating the best evidence available at the time alternatives must be assessed and a decision made will result in better decisions, thereby improving organizational performance.

Figure 5.2 depicts the familiar Shewhart PDSA cycle frequently used in quality improvement efforts in health organizations (Kelly 2003; Institute for Healthcare Improvement 2003; Juran 1989). Although research evidence can be useful in making decisions throughout this cycle, the knowledge base created by the Plan and Study steps—understanding the nature of the problem, the process in which it is embedded, and the effects of any given intervention—can be greatly increased by comparing local data with studies of other organizations.

The generic eight-step decision-making model and the PDSA decision-making approach for improving quality share several strengths. The models help managers systematically identify causes of problems. They provide insights necessary for designing and implementing interventions to improve performance. Each encourages monitoring and evaluation of decisions to continually improve performance over time.

These models also share some important weaknesses. They tend to make improvement processes "inward looking," focusing on information and data that are available or can be generated within the organization. The models place little emphasis on systematic research in other organiza-

FIGURE 5.2
The Shewhart
PDSA Quality
Improvement
Cycle

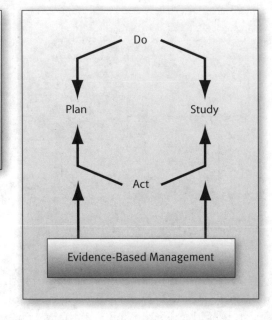

- Plan: Study the process
- Do: Make the changes on a small scale
- Study: Observe the effects
- Act: Identify what was learned

SOURCE: Adapted from Kelly (2003, 32).

tions. Neither model makes use of modern electronic resources to help managers solve problems. Hence, the use of EB management techniques can strengthen these decision-making processes by extending the vision of decision makers beyond their organization's walls, bringing existing evidence into the decision-making process, and providing managers access to the entire spectrum of evidence available on the Internet.

To What Types of Management Questions Can Evidence-Based Management Be Applied?

EB management can be applied to three types of management issues: core business transaction management, operational management, and strategic management. Management questions include those that directly influence the way in which patient care is financed, organized, and delivered, as well as those that are supportive to patient care and those that involve external arrangements among nonclinical personnel (See Table 5.1).

Although EB management techniques can be applied to management decisions regarding core business transactions, research on these issues is not easily available to health services managers. Management decisions regarding core business transactions may be made by trial and error, copying successful processes in other organizations, or seeking technical consultation. On the

TABLE 5.1
Examples of
Management
Questions to
Which EB man-
agement Can
Be Applied

Type of Management Issue	Management Questions
Core Business Transactions	• How can the payer process MD claims for payment more quickly? • How can the health system's information on patient eligibility for benefits be made more accurate? • What methods for paying physician claims achieve speed, convenience, and accuracy requirements?
Operational Management	• How can nurse absenteeism be reduced? • Will decreasing the patient–nurse ratio improve patient outcomes? • Does hospital discharge planning and follow up improve patients' outcomes? • Does hand washing among healthcare workers reduce hospital-acquired infections? • Does basing part of employees' compensation on achievement of unit or team goals improve teamwork and coordination?
Strategic Management	• How do hospital mergers affect administrative costs? • Do hospital–physician joint ventures, such as orthopedic surgery centers, have negative effects on in-hospital surgery? • Does the implementation of an electronic medical record improve the quality of patient care? • Do pay-for-performance incentives substantially improve targeted care processes?

SOURCE: Adapted from Shortell et al. (2000).

other hand, considerable research is available to address many (but not all) operational and strategic issues confronting health services managers. Indeed, systematic reviews exist that summarize research evidence on each of the operational and strategic management questions listed in Table 5.1 at the Agency for Healthcare Research and Quality (www.ahrq.gov/research/), the Cochrane Collaboration Effective Practice and Organization of Care Group (www.epoc.uottawa.ca), and the Cochrane Consumers and Communication Review Group (www.latrobe.edu.au/cochrane) websites. These sites also provide a considerable amount of research regarding organizational structures and processes that may influence patient care processes and patient outcomes.

Applying evidence to the assessment of alternatives and the selection of a "best" alternative is itself a five-step process:

1. Formulating the research question
2. Acquiring the relevant research findings and other types of evidence
3. Assessing the validity, quality, and applicability of the evidence
4. Presenting the evidence in a way that will make it likely that it will be used in the decision process
5. Applying the evidence in decision making

The brief exposition of each step below will illuminate the main features of the approach. (For other more detailed discussions of evidence-based decision making see Muir Gray 2004; Mack, Crawford, and Reed 2004; and Mays, Pope, and Popay 2005).

Formulating the Research Question

The first step is to turn the management question into a research question, framing the issue in a way that will increase the probability of locating useful research studies. This task requires more thought than one may first believe. Often, a very specific management question will have to be broadened to find relevant research, but overly broad, vague, or highly abstract research questions must be avoided. For example, if a manager is interested in knowing the likely effect of implementing a hospitalist program on the cost and quality of care for patients treated for cardiac problems in a suburban Arizona hospital, finding even one study that meets all the inclusion criteria implied by such a narrow, specific question is unlikely. Broadening the management question somewhat (e.g., What is the impact of a hospitalist program on the cost and quality of inpatient care in U.S. community hospitals?) makes it more likely that studies will be found that will be of some value to the hospitalist program implementation decision. However, broadening the question too much (e.g., What is the impact of hospitalists on the healthcare delivery system?) makes it likely that many studies included will not be relevant to the specific issue of interest to the manager. A good guideline for formulating the research question is to incorporate into the question statements that clarify the technique, the setting, and the outcome of interest (see Box 5.1).

Box 5.1
Guidelines for
Formulating an
Appropriate
Research
Question

- What management tool or technique is being considered?
- What is the setting in which the technique would be applied?
- What is the desired managerial process or outcome?

Acquiring Research Evidence

Evidence relevant to the management research question can be obtained from a wide array of sources; colleagues, consultants, and known experts are frequent sources of evidence. Many managers will find it helpful to use the Internet to locate research articles. Health organizations that have made significant investments in knowledge management may have libraries, trained librarians and webmasters, intranet information resources, or an in-house management decision-support system. The vast majority of managers will not have such resources, but will be limited to what they can find on the open Internet.

Two general approaches can be used to acquire research evidence via the open Internet:

1. Searching websites that provide access to systematic reviews or meta-analyses. For example, the Effective Practice and Organization of Care (EPOC) group within the Cochrane Library as mentioned above may provide insight.
2. Searching bibliographic databases such as MEDLINE, PubMed, or Google Scholar for published and unpublished primary studies of relevance to the research question (see Box 5.2). For example using the search terms "hospitalist," "cost," and "quality" to search the Scholar Google database produced over 60 citations, many of which appeared to be qualitative or quantitative research studies. One of those articles was co-authored by one of us (Coffman and Rundall 2005).

Box 5.2 Resources for Health Services Management Research

Agency for Healthcare Research and Quality:
www.ahrq.gov/research

Effective Practice and Organization of Care Group:
www.epoc.uottawa.ca

Consumers and Communication Review Group:
www.latrobe.edu.au/cochrane

Center for Health Management Research:
http://depts.washington.edu/chmr/research

PubMed: www.ncbi.nlm.nih.gov/entrez/query.fcgi?db=PubMed

MEDLINE: www.nlm.nih.gov/databases/databases_medline.html

Google Scholar: http://scholar.google.com

A research synthesis of a large number of primary research articles is especially useful to decision makers since the authors of the synthesis have already made an attempt to assess the quality of the evidence and to draw out the conclusions that are supported by the evidence. Once relevant articles have been found, they may be electronically stored and, if desired, printed out to make them easier to read and assess.

What types of evidence can be incorporated in EB management? This issue has caused considerable debate in the EB management literature. Some analysts have argued that EB management should follow the lead of evidence-based medicine and rely upon evidence syntheses, which are systematic reviews of the evidence from studies of the effects of a particular policy or managerial intervention.

Critics of this rather restrictive definition of evidence point out that relatively few evidence syntheses are available on issues of concern to health services managers, that the standard procedures for carrying out systematic reviews dismiss many useful studies as methodologically weak, and that from a managerial perspective the knowledge and insights gained from qualitative case studies, expert opinion, and personal experience should be considered evidence (Davies and Nutley 1999; Bero and Jadad 1997; Mays, Pope, and Popay 2005; Pawson et al. 2005). This issue is far from resolved as it involves the age-old debate over the need for balance between rigor and relevance in applied research.

As Ham recently pointed out, dismissing the relevance of systematic reviews and giving personal experience and other kinds of intelligence equal standing with the evidence generated by formal research studies runs the risk of "throwing the baby out with the bath water" (Ham 2005). A compromise approach may be to relax the criteria for the inclusion of studies and extend search strategies beyond established databases (Ham 2005). Moreover, researchers and managers must remember that the principles of EB management as described at the outset of this article explicitly incorporate both rigorous research as well as experiential judgment and research studies conducted with smaller samples and weaker designs than would be desirable. The point of the EB management approach is to create an expectation that managers will seek the best research evidence available at the time a decision is made, and to incorporate this evidence with other sources of information, such as expert opinion and personal experience in the decision-making process.

Assessing the Quality of the Evidence

Managers must have some minimal competency in assessing management research, critical appraisal skills that will enable them to judge the quality of the evidence available. Ideally, managers should have, or have available to them, competency to assess:

- Strength of the research design
- Study context and setting
- Sample sizes of the study groups
- Control for confounding factors
- Reliability and validity of the measurements
- Methods and procedures used
- Justification of the conclusions
- Study sponsorship
- Consistency of the findings with other studies

In many cases, these issues will be addressed in the research report itself. For example, in the Coffman and Rundall evidence synthesis of studies of the effect of hospitalists on hospital costs and quality of care, 21 studies were identified that met minimal inclusion and exclusion search criteria. Still, these studies varied significantly in their overall research designs (e.g., experimental design with randomized control group versus quasi-experimental designs without randomization); types of comparison groups used in the quasi-experimental studies (e.g., concurrent versus historical); the size of the intervention and control/comparison groups; the statistical control for confounding factors; and the length of time over which the intervention was operative before evaluation data were collected. To understand the findings from these studies, these important differences in the strengths of the studies, and hence in the quality of the evidence, were incorporated in the synthesis. At a minimum, managers should be aware of the importance of assessing these aspects of research studies and be able to evaluate the extent to which they have been addressed in any given primary research study or research synthesis.

Presenting the Evidence

Managers and researchers should present evidence to the decision-making process in a way that is timely, brief, avoids technical jargon, provides clear descriptions of the questions addressed, incorporates the context of the research and findings, offers an assessment of the strength of the evidence, gives the results and implications for practice, and is easy to access (see Box 5.3). The Coffman and Rundall (2005) synthesis attempted to present the evidence found in multiple studies in a way that would be understandable to managers and other nonspecialists in the field. The 21 studies were organized into groups based on strength of research design and methods. Simple tables were used showing how many of the 21 studies in each group demonstrated reduction in resource use (e.g., lower total costs or charges), improvement in measures of quality of care (e.g., lower readmission rate), and increase in patient satisfaction (e.g., self-reported satisfaction with patient care experience).

Box 5.3
Guidelines for
Presentation
of Evidence

- Present timely evidence.
- Be brief.
- Avoid technical jargon.
- Provide clear descriptions of the questions addressed.
- Incorporate the context of the research and findings.
- Offer an assessment of the strength of the evidence.
- Give the results and implications for practice.
- Make the presentation easy to access.

The Coffman and Rundall article is not offered as a "best practice" of how to present evidence to health services managers. Indeed, publishing a briefer version in a journal explicitly marketed to managers would have increased its reach. However, we believe that managers, clinicians, and patients who searched for and found this article would have understood the findings. Managers and clinicians in hospitals and physician organizations could have easily incorporated these findings, including the qualifications proposed by the authors, into their assessment of the likely effects of adopting a hospitalist program.

Applying the Evidence to the Decision

Getting health services organization decision makers to use evidence may be the most challenging step. Most organizations today do not have the incentives or capabilities necessary for routinely using evidence in decision making. Substantial staff time is often required to ensure an adequate deliberative process. Opportunity costs are associated with disseminating and discussing the implications of research findings for a particular decision in a given organization. Ego costs to managers and others who feel their preferences are challenged by the evidence might be incurred.

The multiple ways in which research evidence assists the decision-making process are poorly understood. Many users demand that the available evidence have immediate, instrumental use for a particular decision, but often the available research evidence cannot be used in that way. Rather, the evidence is better used to increase the decision maker's enlightenment regarding the decision issue by increasing the manager's understanding of the nature of a problem; opening up communication among managers and other stakeholders; enabling the manager to generate creative solutions; and enhancing the manager's ability to estimate the likely effects of each alternative solution to a problem. These are important, but under appreciated, contributions of the evidence-based approach to decision making.

In fact, the same body of evidence can be used for instrumental and enlightenment purposes by organizations in different stages of a

decision process. For example, the Coffman and Rundall evidence synthesis on the effects of hospitalists on hospital costs and quality of care
was presented to representatives of several health systems that are members of the Center for Health Management Research (CHMR). This
presentation increased the representatives' awareness of the availability
of the various studies and their findings. More instrumental use was made
of the synthesis by one of the CHMR member health systems who invited
a coauthor of the study to present the results to over 60 middle- and sen-
ior-level managers as part of a seminar on evidence-based management.
The findings from the synthesis were incorporated in on going discussions about whether and how to implement hospitalist programs in the
system's hospitals. At another CHMR health system, the results of the
synthesis were presented at a board of directors' meeting and contributed
directly to the system's decision to implement hospitalist programs in
two of its hospitals.

A Study of the Use of Evidence in Decision Making by Health Services Managers in the United States

Kovner (2005) recently conducted a study designed to identify and explore
factors associated with knowledge transfer between researchers and managers of health systems. The research focused on managers of five health
systems and four types of decisions. The decision issues were: selecting the
indicators for assessing the success of diabetes management programs;
strengthening the relationship between budgeting procedures and strategic
priorities; selecting the operational metrics to include in managerial dashboards, and adapting compensation systems for managers of physician performance. The study methodology included 68 interviews of managers of
17 nonprofit health systems located in regions throughout the United States.
Of these interviews, 56 were with managers of five health systems that were
members of the CHMR. The other 12 interviews were with managers in
12 health systems similar in size and sponsorship to one or more of the five
CHMR health systems. In each interview, each manager was asked a series
of questions to gain an understanding of whether they used evidence in
decision making about each of the four issues described above, and how evidence was used to make decisions in their organization. Specifically, the
managers were asked:

- Can you tell us about a recent decision that you are or were part of making?
- What process did the team working on the decision use to find evidence?
- In what respect was this a typical process, or not, for this type of decision?
- How do you assess if the evidence is of high quality, relevant, and
  applicable?

- What are three professional journals, websites, or other publications you find most useful in making decisions?

As in the Canadian and United Kingdom studies of evidence use by health services managers, U.S. managers reported little use of the evidence-based approach as described above for decision making. None of the 68 managers interviewed mentioned using evidence from management research to make strategic decisions. The journals that managers found useful were not research journals, or if they were research journals, they were not management journals. Journals cited included the *Harvard Business Review*, *Modern Healthcare*, *Health Affairs*, and *The New England Journal of Medicine*. Twenty-two websites were mentioned as useful, including those of the Agency for Health Care Research and Quality (www.ahrq.gov), Centers for Medicare & Medicaid Services (cms.hhs.gov), the Institute of Healthcare Improvement (www.ihi.org), and the Joint Commission on the Accreditation of Healthcare Organizations (www.jcaho.org). The data from this study suggest that there is a good deal of similarity between U.S. health services managers and their Canadian and British counterparts.

Interestingly, when asked, "How do you feel that your organization's culture promotes your use of evidence in decision making?" respondents gave generally positive comments. All 15 of the 15 respondents in the five health systems that were specifically asked this question spoke positively that their system's culture promoted the use of evidence in decision making. The apparent contradiction between the reported non-use of EB management and organizational cultures favorable to the use of evidence in decision making is rooted in the managers' working definition of "evidence." As in Canada and the United Kingdom, the definition of evidence among health services managers differs from that used by most health services researchers (Canadian Health Services Research Foundation 2004). Many respondents indicated that they used evidence in making decisions, but what they referred to as evidence was frequently their own experience, anecdotes that had been communicated to them, information from Internet sites, and advice from consultants and advisory organizations such as the Health Care Advisory Board. None of the managers interviewed reported that in their organizations the evidentiary process for strategic decision making was regularly reviewed or that there was formal oversight of the deliberative process.

In further analyzing the data to identify ideas and strategies that might be used to increase the use of EB management, Kovner (2005) identified four factors that respondents suggested may influence use of management research in health systems:

- External demands for performance accountability
- An accountability structure for knowledge transfer

- A questioning organizational culture
- Participation in management research

From these findings, we recommend strategies for increasing the use of evidence-based decision making among health services managers.

Strategies to Increase the Use of Evidence-Based Management

External Demands for Performance Accountability

The increasing demands for accountability by external organizations have conflicting effects on the use of EB management. Managers reported that their systems were increasingly expected and/or required to meet process and outcome performance targets set by purchasers, quality improvement organizations, and public and private regulatory groups. These external organizations, such as the Joint Commission on the Accreditation of Health Organizations, the Centers for Medicare & Medicaid Services, the National Quality Forum, the Leapfrog Group, and national and regional pay-for-performance programs, are increasingly identifying healthcare patient care process and outcome criteria and setting performance standards for health systems. Health system managers clearly recognize the strategic importance of the recognition and rewards offered by these external organizations, and in many cases such external pressures for accountability increase the use of EB management. However, in other cases managers are concerned that motivation to search for and use research evidence in their quality improvement efforts is undermined by the focus on quality improvement processes, outcomes, and performance targets set by external agencies. One health system manager expressed this concern in the following way:

In the past, before there were so many requirements for data reporting, we had a different process for setting performance indicators. We looked at the literature for the right thing to do, and then we met with committees of physicians and nurses and asked them what was important....Today, however, there is so much demand for publicly reported data that we don't choose which areas to try to develop and improve dashboards and scorecards. We respond to demand.

In environments where external stakeholders are setting health systems' performance criteria and standards, we suggest that managers clearly link evidence searching and application to the development of organizational structures and processes that improve organizational performance on the externally set criteria, in effect marrying evidence-based medicine and evidence-based management to deliver the right treatment to the right patient, for the right condition, at the right time. In this way the strategic importance of EB management can be established and enhanced over time as the use of research evidence is seen to contribute to the design of more effective processes for delivering care that meets externally set performance targets. If EB management is not perceived to be strategically important to a health system, few resources will be devoted to it.

An Accountability Structure for Knowledge Transfer

Formalizing the responsibility structure for dissemination and use of evidence focuses and increases the impact of knowledge transfer. If no one is responsible for a function, it is unlikely that the function will be performed effectively in a complex, large healthcare organization. To be a priority goal, dissemination and use of management research must be seen as consistent with and as contributing to the organizational goals of the leadership. On the other hand, the lack of an accountability structure contributes to a casual approach to searching for evidence that typically relies on convenient sources and minimal effort. For example, one health system manager reported:

> I get evidence from two sources: conversations with other people in the healthcare industry, and my past professional experience.

Unfortunately, health systems do not designate managers as being responsible and accountable for knowledge transfer or for assessing research evidence as part of their decision-making process. Moreover, at the present time metrics are lacking to assess the benefits of obtaining better evidence for management decision making. Clearly, the use of EB management would increase if health systems assigned responsibility for knowledge management to individuals or teams within the organization. A parallel strategy is to fix management responsibility for review of deliberative processes as part of the regular process of strategic decision making.

A Questioning Organizational Culture

A questioning culture affects the amount and speed of knowledge transfer between producers, disseminators, and targets of EB management research. Health systems that support evidence-based decision making have cultures that recognize that encouraging questioning behavior among managers can lessen future problems that arise out of hasty and insufficiently considered decisions (see Box 5.4). However, challenging decisions and introducing research evidence into problem-solving discussions can cause anxiety among managers, creating a sense that managerial judgment and expertise are perceived by colleagues as inadequate or not trustworthy. As a health system respondent put it:

On a philosophical basis, people tend to agree [about the desirability of evidence-based management] When it comes to actually doing the work though, you start getting push back.

We suggest several strategies for building a questioning culture. Managers can participate in research "rounds," management research journal clubs, or research seminars led by internal managers or researchers from academic or other research institutions. Managers can routinely be asked by senior leaders to analyze the results of past operational and strategic decisions, including comparing their systems' performance with findings from research on other organizations. Staff development programs can be conducted to help institutionalize evidence-based decision making and enhance managers' abilities to find, assess, and apply research findings. Managers' compensation can be linked to metrics related to obtaining and using relevant evidence in decision making and sharing evidence with key stakeholders. Finally, we suggest that health systems develop organizational guidelines for decision making that require an assessment of available research evidence.

- Organize research rounds, management research journal clubs, and research seminars.
- Analyze the results of past operational and strategic decisions, including comparing the systems' performance with findings from research on other organizations.
- Conduct staff development programs to enhance managers' abilities to find, assess, and apply research findings.
- Link compensation to metrics related to obtaining and using relevant evidence in decision making and sharing evidence with key stakeholders.
- Develop guidelines for decision making that require an assessment of research evidence.

Box 5.4
Building a
Questioning
Culture

Participation in Management Research

Research dissemination, use, and impact will be affected by the level of participation of health system management in knowledge transfer. Lavis and others (2003) found that research transfer often required interactive engagement, as it is a very time-consuming and skill-intensive process. They stress the importance of developing uptake skills for research among target audiences. In the Kovner study, managers that conducted their own studies, focus groups, or market assessments were more supportive of evidence-based decision making. However, these managers had limited evidence-searching and appraisal skills. None of the health systems employed specialists in knowledge management. Access to resources such as the Cochrane Collaboration website or even management journals was limited. Clearly, familiarity with research and with the skills and technologic apparatus associated with health services research are important factors driving the use of evidence in decision making. In some cases, these shortcomings can be overcome through the use of consulting or specialized research services. In the case of one health system:

> We developed a strategic plan for our heart services. Part of that was gaining an understanding of the minds of consumers in the local market....We used a national company to do a random study....This was an empirical work; it was a conjoint study. It gave us longitudinal ideas and information about our primary market. The national company asked questions that were our questions. We hired a company that does consumer research and we told them what we wanted to know.

Several strategies can increase health systems managers' research capability and actual participation in management research:

- Management training in EB management;
- Investing internal funds in management research projects;
- Partnering with research organizations, such as survey firms and academic research centers; and
- Implementing information technology and knowledge management systems.

To put in perspective the findings reported above, we introduce some key ideas from the work of Shortell and his colleagues (2000) on the key success factors for clinical integration in health services. Shortell and his colleagues identified four organizational dimensions (strategic, structural, cultural, and technical) that influence delivery systems' ability to achieve significant organizational change, such as clinical integration. We adapted their framework and have applied it to our findings about the use of EB management in health systems.

The Strategic Dimension

The strategic dimension emphasizes that significant organizational change—such as the adoption of EB management practices—must focus on strategically important issues facing the health system. The implication is that to be widely used in health systems, EB management must be seen by health system managers as a core strategic priority of the system. Our finding regarding the influence of external demands for performance accountability—a key strategic issue for health systems—on managers' support for EB management is consistent with this dimension.

The Structural Dimension

The structural dimension refers to the overall structure of the system to support EB management, including the use of designated committees, task forces, and individuals identified as responsible for implementing and diffusing EB management practices. Our finding about the need for an accountability structure for knowledge transfer fits well within this dimension.

The Cultural Dimension

The cultural dimension refers to the beliefs, norms, values, and behaviors of people in the health system who may either support or oppose EB management. Our findings regarding the importance of having a questioning culture as a precondition for EB management are consistent with this dimension.

The Technical Dimension

The technical dimension refers to the extent to which people have the necessary knowledge, training, and skills to practice EB management and the extent to which they have access to information technology and other technological assets. Again, our findings with regard to the importance of managers' having research skills, experience in performing research, and the critical appraisal skills necessary to assess research evidence performed by others is consistent with this dimension.

As Shortell and colleagues (2000) argue, to achieve a high degree of organizational change in core processes such as the integration of clinical services or the use of research evidence in management decision making, health systems "must attend to all four dimensions simultaneously and attempt to align them with each other" (p. 140). In Table 5.2 we have suggested what happens when one or another dimension is missing.

When the strategic dimension is missing, no important decisions are made using research evidence. When efforts are made to practice EB management, they have little effect because they are not directed at the strategic priorities of the system.

When the structural dimension is missing, sporadic, isolated efforts to incorporate research evidence in decision making may occur, but little systemwide use of evidence-based decision making is present. This is because no one is accountable for diffusing these practices throughout the system and few appropriate committees or task forces train and disseminate the concepts and techniques of evidence-based decision making.

When the cultural component is missing, efforts to introduce evidence-based decision making quickly wither and fade away because the organizational culture does not support EB management. People do not

TABLE 5.2
Effect of Organizational Components on Use of EB management

External Demands for Performance Accountability (Strategic Dimension)	Accountability Structure for Knowledge Transfer (Structural Dimension)	Questioning Culture (Cultural Dimension)	Participation in Management Research (Technical Dimension)	Result
absent	present	present	present	No significant use of research evidence on anything really important
present	absent	present	present	Inability to acquire research evidence and disseminate it throughout the system
present	present	absent	present	Small, intermittent use of evidence in decision making; no lasting impact
present	present	present	absent	Frustration and false starts in attempts to incorporate evidence in decision making
present	present	present	present	Lasting systemwide adoption of evidence-based management

☐ = present   ■ = absent

SOURCE: Adapted from Shortell et al. (2000).

believe evidence-based decision making will produce better decisions, and it is not rewarded by the organization.

Absence of the technical dimension results in frustration and false starts in attempts to implement EB management because managers do not have the necessary training in the principles of evidence-based decision making, evidence searching, and research appraisal, and they may not have access to needed Internet and other resources.

This interpretation of the findings may indicate why EB management is so little used, and suggests that a concerted effort will be required to change the situation. Only when all four dimensions are simultaneously made more supportive of EB management and aligned with each other will sustainable progress occur.

Conclusion

The extent to which evidence-based decision making remains outside the repertoire of many health services managers is reflected in the way management mistakes are handled in most organizations and by instances of major decisions being made without regard to existing evidence that bears on the issue.

The rationale for using an evidence-based approach to managing health services organizations mirrors the rationale for evidence-based medicine. The movement toward evidence-based clinical practice was prompted by the observation of unexplained wide variations in clinical practice patterns, by the poor uptake of therapies of known effectiveness, and by the persistent use of treatments and technologies known to be ineffective. These problems are also common in managerial practice in healthcare organizations.

The sense of urgency associated with improving the quality of medical care does not exist with respect to improving the quality of management decision making. One reason for this complacency is that instances of overuse, underuse, and misuse of management tactics and strategies receive far less attention and are much more difficult to document than their clinical equivalents. Surely, mistakes of judgment that result in irrefutable harm to people, significant financial loss, or profound organizational change may motivate public and private inquiries into "how could this have happened?" For example, the failed merger of the hospitals owned by Stanford University and the University of California at San Francisco cost both institutions a combined $176 million over a 29-month period and stimulated considerable public discussion of the reasons for the failure of the merger (Russell 2000). However, the visibility of the Stanford–UCSF hospital fiasco stands in stark contrast to the way most management mistakes are handled. Relatively few ineffective or harmful management decisions are acknowledged, examined, and used as the source of organizational learning (Hofmann 2005; Jones 2005; Russell and Greenspan 2005). Moreover, the fact that a merger of two highly rated hospitals with close ties to world-renowned universities could proceed in spite of a substantial body of research that was available at the time that raised serious concerns about that type of merger (Bogue et al. 1995; Alexander, Halpern, and Lee 1996; Brooks and Jones 1997; Conner et al. 1997) serves as a vivid and painful reminder of a management quality chasm in health services organizations. A substantial gap exists between what is known about many management questions and what health managers do. We must close this gap.

Note

1. The Healthcare Leadership Alliance comprises the American College of Healthcare Executives, American College of Physician Executives,

American Organization of Nurse Executives, Healthcare Financial Management Association, Healthcare Information and Management Systems Society, Medical Group Management Association, and the American College of Medical Practice Executives.

Acknowledgment

The authors gratefully acknowledge the assistance of Chris Kovner, Juliana Tilemma, and Erica Foldy, and of course the managers whom Kovner interviewed in the collection of information used in the preparation of this article. We would also like to acknowledge the financial support of the Center for Health Management Research in conducting the research reported here.

References

Agency for Healthcare Research and Quality (AHRQ). 2006a. National Guideline Clearinghouse. [Online resource; modified 10/10/05; retrieved 10/13/05.] www.guideline.gov.

———. 2006b. Research Findings [Online resource; retrieved 10/21/05.] www.ahrq.gov/research.

Alexander, J. A., M. T. Halpern, and S-Y. D. Lee. 1996. "The Short-Term Effects of Merger on Hospital Operations." *Health Services Research* 30 (6): 827–47.

Axelson, R. 1998. "Towards an Evidence-Based Health Care Management." *International Journal of Health Planning and Management* 13: 307–17.

Bero, L. A., and A. R. Jadad. 1997. "How Consumers and Policymakers Can Use Systematic Reviews for Decision Making." *Annals of Internal Medicine* 127 (127): 37–42.

Bogue, R. J., S. M. Shortell, M. W. Sohn, L. M. Manheim, G. Bazzoli, and C. Chan. 1995. "Hospital Reorganization After Merger." *Medical Care* 33 (7): 676–86.

Brooks, G. R., and V. G. Jones. 1997. "Hospital Mergers and Market Overlap." *Health Services Research* 31 (6): 701–22.

Brownson, R. C., E. A. Baker, T. L. Leet, and K. N. Gillespie. 2003. *Evidence-Based Public Health*. Oxford: Oxford University Press.

Canadian Health Services Research Foundation. 2000. *Health Services Research and Evidence-Based Decision Making, 7*. Ottawa, Canada: Health Services Research Foundation.

———. 2004. *What Counts? Interpreting Evidence-Based Decision-Making for Management and Policy*. Ottawa, Canada: Health Services Research Foundation.

———. 2005. *Conceptualizing and Combining Evidence for Health System Guidance*. Ottawa, Canada: Health Services Research Foundation.

Clancy, C., and K. Cronin. 2005. "Evidence-Based Decision Making: Global Evidence, Local Decisions." *Health Affairs* 24 (1): 151–62.

Cochrane Effective Practice and Organization of Care Group. 2006. [Online resource; updated 5/24/04; retrieved 10/13/05] http://www.epoc.uottawa.ca/

Cochrane Consumers and Communication Review Group. 2006 [Online resource; updated 10/12/05; retrieved 10/21/05] http://www.latrobe.edu.au/cochrane/

Coffman, J., and T. G. Rundall. 2005. "The Impact of Hospitalists on the Cost and Quality of Inpatient Care in the United States: A Research Synthesis." *Medical Care Research and Review* 62 (4): 379–406.

Conner, R. A., R. D. Feldman, B. E. Dowd, and T. A. Radcliff. 1997. "Which Types of Hospital Mergers Save Money?" *Health Affairs* 16 (6): 62–74.

Davies, H. T. O., and S. M. Nutley. 1999. "The Rise and Rise of Evidence in Health Care." *Public Money and Management* (Jan–Mar): 9–16.

Donaldson, C., M. Mugford, and L. Vale. 2002. *Evidence-Based Health Economics.* London: BMJ Books.

Eddy, D. M. 2005. "Evidence-Based Medicine: A Unified Approach." *Health Affairs* 24 (1): 9–17.

Friedland, D. J., ed. 1998. *Evidence-Based Medicine: A Framework for Clinical Practice.* Stamford, CT: Appleton & Lange.

Fox, D. 2005. "Evidence of Evidence-Based Health Policy: The Politics of Systematic Reviews in Coverage Decision." *Health Affairs* 24 (1): 114–22.

Geyman, J. P., R. A. Deyo, and S. D. Ramsey. 2000. *Evidence-Based Clinical Practice: Concepts and Approaches.* Boston: Butterworth and Heinemann.

Greenhalgh, T., G. Robert, F. Macfarlane, P. Bate, and O. Kyriakidou. 2004. "Diffusion of Innovations in Service Organizations: Systematic Review and Recommendations." *The Milbank Quarterly* 82 (4): 581–629.

Ham, C. 2005. "Don't Throw the Baby Out With the Bath Water" (commentary). *Journal of Health Services Research and Policy* 10 (S1): 51–52.

Hatcher, S., and M. Oakley-Browne. 2005. *Evidence-Based Mental Health.* London: Churchill Livingston.

Healthcare Leadership Alliance. 2005. "Competency Directory." [Online document; retrieved 12/13/05.] www.healthcareleadershipalliance.org/directory.cfm.

Hofmann, P. B. 2005. "Acknowledging and Examining Management Mistakes." In *Management Mistakes in Healthcare: Identification, Correction, and Prevention*, edited by P. B. Hofmann and F. Perry, 3–27. Cambridge: Cambridge University Press.

Hofmann, P. B., and F. Perry. 2005. *Management Mistakes in Healthcare: Identification, Correction, and Prevention.* Cambridge: Cambridge University Press.

Institute for Healthcare Improvement. 2003. "Breakthrough Series Collaboratives." [Online information; retrieved 06/06/02.] www.ihi.org/ihi.

Jones, W. J. 2005. "Identifying, Classifying and Disclosing Mistakes." In *Management Mistakes in Healthcare: Identification, Correction, and Prevention*, edited by P. B. Hofmann and F. Perry, 40–73. Cambridge: Cambridge University Press.

Juran, J. M. 1989. *Juran on Leadership for Quality: An Executive Handbook.* New York: The Free Press.

Kelly, D. L. 2003. *Applying Quality Management in Healthcare: A Process for Improvement.* Chicago: Health Administration Press.

Kovner, A. R. 2005. "Factors Associated with Use of Management Research by Health Systems." Unpublished report for the Center for Health Management Research, University of Washington, Seattle.

Kovner, A. R., J. J. Elton, and J. Billings. 2000. "Transforming Health Management: An Evidence-Based Approach." *Frontiers of Health Services Management* 16 (4): 3–25.

Lavis, J., H. Davies, A. Oxman, J.-L. Denis, K. Golden-Biddle, and E. Ferlie. 2005. "Towards Systematic Reviews That Inform Health Care Management and Policy-Making." *Journal of Health Services Research and Policy* 10 (S1): 35–48.

Lavis, J. N., D. Robertson, J. M. Woodside, C. B. McLeod, J. Abelson, and The Knowledge Transfer Group. 2003. "How Can Research Organizations More Effectively Transfer Research Knowledge to Decision Makers?" *The Milbank Quarterly* 81 (2): 221–48.

Lavis, J. N., S. E. Ross, J. E. Hurley, J. M. Hohenadel, G. L. Stoddart, C. A. Woodward, and J. Abelson. 2002. "Examining the Role of Health Services Research in Public Policy Making." *Milbank Quarterly* 80 (1): 125–53.

Lomas, J. 2000. "Using 'Linkage and Exchange' to Move Research into Policy at a Canadian Foundation." *Health Affairs* 19 (3): 236–40.

Mack, K. E., M. A. Crawford, and M. C. Reed. 2004. *Decision Making for Improved Performance.* Chicago: Health Administration Press.

Mays N., C. Pope, and J. Popay. 2005. "Systematically Reviewing Qualitative and Quantitative Evidence to Inform Management and Policy-Making in the Health Field." *Journal of Health Services Research and Policy* 10 (S1): 6–20.

Muir Gray, J. A. 2004. *Evidence-Based Health Care: How to Make Health Policy and Management Decisions.* New York: Churchill Livingston.

National Center for Healthcare Leadership. 2004. Health Leadership Competency Model, version 2.0, 1–9. Chicago: National Center for Healthcare Leadership.

Pawson, R., T. Greenhalgh, G. Harvey, and K. Walshe. 2005. "Realist Review—A New Method of Systematic Review Designed for Complex

Policy Interventions." *Journal of Health Services Research and Policy* 10 (S1): 21–34.

Robbins, S. P., and D. A. DeCenzo. 2004. *Fundamentals of Management: Essential Concepts and Applications*, 4th edition. Upper Saddle River, NJ: Pearson Prentice Hall.

Russell, J. A., and B. Greenspan. 2005. "Correcting and Preventing Management Mistakes." In *Management Mistakes in Healthcare: Identification, Correction, and Prevention*, edited by P. B. Hofmann and F. Perry, 84–102. Cambridge: Cambridge University Press.

Russell, S. 2000. "$176 Million Tab on Failed Hospital Merger." *San Francisco Chronicle*, December 14.

Sackett, D. L., W. M. Rosenberg, J. A. Gray, R. B. Haynes, and W. S. Richardson. 1996. "Evidence-Based Medicine: What It Is and What It Isn't." *British Medical Journal* 312 (7023): 71–72.

Sackett, D. L., S. E. Straus, W. S. Richardson, W. Rosenberg, and R. B. Haynes. 2000. *Evidence-Based Medicine: How to Practice and Teach EBM*, 2nd edition. New York: Churchill Livingston.

Sheldon, T. 2005. "Making Evidence Synthesis More Useful for Management and Policy-Making." *Journal of Health Services Research and Policy* 10 (S1): 1–4.

Shojania, K. G., and J. M. Grimshaw. 2005. "Evidence-Based Quality Improvement: The State of the Science." *Health Affairs* 24 (1): 138–50.

Shortell, S. M., R. R. Gillies, D. A. Anderson, K. M. Erickson, and J. B. Mitchell. 2000. *Remaking Health Care in America*, 2nd edition. San Francisco: Jossey-Bass.

Shortell, S. 2001. "A Time for Concerted Action." *Frontiers of Health Services Management* 18 (1): 33–46.

Stewart, R. 2002. *Evidence-Based Management: A Practical Guide for Health Professionals*. Abingdon, UK: Radcliffe Medical Press.

Walshe, K., and T. Rundall. 2001. "Evidence-Based Management: From Theory to Practice in Health Care." *The Milbank Quarterly* 79 (3): 429–47.

EVIDENCE-BASED MANAGEMENT RECONSIDERED: 18 MONTHS LATER

Thomas G. Rundall and Anthony R. Kovner

This is a follow-up to the previous chapter.

Since the publication of our article "Evidence-Based Management Reconsidered" (Kovner and Rundall 2006) we have continued to discuss the issues it raised. The basic arguments we brought forth continue to seem valid, and we are pleased to observe the spread of EB management to the non-health sector through the work of several authors.[1] We would like to continue the dialog here.

In our report, we argued that sustainable progress can occur only when all the strategic, structural, cultural, and technical organizational dimensions support EB management and are aligned with each other. We realize that changing fundamental aspects of managers' work and working styles is difficult, but we were surprised at how much actually needed to change. We learned that managers typically do not research management issues nor use research evidence in decision making. However, we found that younger managers may be more likely to access research evidence because of their facility with electronic databases and the Web. Why don't large health systems fund more management research? What would incent large health systems to support management research and encourage use of research evidence in decision making? What are the costs and benefits of collecting better evidence to inform important management decisions?

Apparently, managers (and consultants) do not see the need for management research in improving quality of care, patient safety, and other aspects of hospital and health system operations—either because they don't recognize the need, don't understand the business case, or aren't motivated or expected to use research-based evidence in their decision making. As EB management proponents, we could strengthen our case by researching what happens when managers use and do not use EB management.[2]

In the *Frontiers* article (see Chapter 5), we suggested a five-step approach to EB management: (1) formulating the research question; (2) acquiring the relevant research findings and other types of evidence; (3) assessing the validity, quality, and applicability of the evidence; (4) presenting the evidence in a way that will make its use in the decision process likely; and (5) applying the evidence in decision making. Where possible in this volume, we've added a sixth step, evaluating the results.

Other researchers have suggested models that incorporate more or fewer steps in the managerial decision-making process. For example, Daft and Marcic (2006) suggest six: recognition of decision requirement, diagnosis and analysis of causes, development of alternatives, selection of desired alternative, implementation of the selected alternative, and evaluation and feedback. The Shewhart PDSA Quality Improvement Cycle approach has four steps: plan, do, study, and act.

Unlike other models, ours is specifically designed to incorporate research evidence in the decision-making process. The number of specific steps is less important than the spirit of the EB management approach, which stresses making a good faith effort to examine existing relevant research, and, when necessary, conducting original research to inform important decisions.

EB management techniques help managers learn to be diligent and consistent in their decision making. Although our model makes it appear as if one moves neatly from step to step, this isn't the case. The steps simply provide a structure for working on a proposed management intervention or evaluation. They overlap, and one may have to return to earlier steps or work on several steps simultaneously as the problem-solving work unfolds. Flexibility is important. Information gathering occurs in all steps, from problem identification to implementation of a solution. New information may force a manager to redefine a problem. Proposed solutions may prove to be unworkable, requiring decision makers to identify new ones. The EB management process is usually not linear; and, under certain circumstances, some steps may even be combined, abbreviated, or eliminated, as demonstrated in several of the case studies later in this book.

The steps of any decision-making process are not completely rational. Managers must reflect upon the biases they bring to the table in seeking and weighing evidence. In clinical medicine, perhaps 15 percent of a doctor's diagnoses may be inaccurate, for reasons not entirely clear, according to noted physician-author Jerome Groopman (2007). This batting average certainly applies to management diagnoses as well. In fact, Groopman cites alarming evidence that the worse radiologists perform, the more convinced they are that they are right. Misplaced confidence (or at least a persona cultivated to convey confidence) may characterize managers as well; the danger is that other people, especially subordinates, will not question the assertions of a supremely confident superior.

Groopman suggests that physicians can easily be led astray by seeing a set of circumstances from only one perspective. He lists the following types of bias:

- Attribution error—discrediting data from a "tainted" source
- Availability error—basing a decision on the most recent experience, even though it bears little relation to past circumstances

- Search satisfaction error—stopping the search for an answer as soon as a satisfactory solution is found
- Confirmation bias—selecting only the parts of the information that confirm an initial judgment
- Diagnostic momentum—being unable to change one's mind about a diagnosis, despite considerable uncertainty
- Commission bias—"doing something" rather than nothing, even if the evidence says sit tight

Inattention and hurry take over for managers as well as for physicians, and many managers do not routinely think through such potential cognitive pitfalls. Groopman urges that physicians recognize and understand their own biases as they approach a decision. He also encourages patients to speak up with physicians. We offer similar advice to managers, particularly those with less experience, who must speak up and be encouraged to do so by senior managers.

Some colleagues argue that EB management appears to be an attempt to breathe new life into the classical/rational approach to decision making, which has been rejected by many scholars as too prescriptive and not applicable in most real-world decision-making situations. We recognize that there are many ways to conceptualize organizational decision making. The classical/rational perspective is prescriptive, and recent organizational scholarship suggests that there is a good deal of real-world use of the approach, particularly for routine organizational decisions.

Other perspectives on decision making, such as the administrative and political perspectives, are more descriptive and de-emphasize the role of research evidence in decision making. We believe that regardless of the decision-making perspective one is using, the use of better evidence, admittedly at a cost, can improve the decision.

Like all decision-making tools (e.g., Pareto analysis, decision trees, force-field analysis, linear programming), the EB management process is prescriptive, inasmuch as it describes activities and tasks that must be performed in order to achieve a desired objective. If a manager wants to use evidence in a decision-making process, the EB management model provides a useful framework for thinking through and doing the necessary tasks. It does not prescribe the kind of evidence, how to obtain it, or what decisions should be made. As readers will observe in the case studies, "evidence" covers a lot of intellectual territory.

Many healthcare managers reacted to our article with some mixture of enthusiasm and uncertainty. Some said, essentially, "I like what you wrote, and I like the idea of EB management, but how much of this should I implement, in what ways, in my organization?" We did not and cannot offer precise answers to such questions. We do suggest that these managers spend some more time focusing on their strategic decision-making process—

developing structures that establish accountability for using an EB management approach, building a questioning culture, and improving the training of the managerial workforce in applying the EB management approach.

With experience, best practices will emerge, and we will need mechanisms for sharing them. One such mechanism already in place is an EB management website (http://evidence-basedmanagement.com), which includes a blog through which managers can share experiences.

Finally, we hypothesize that healthcare managers who make decisions based on better evidence work in organizations that, in the long run, will be shown to provide better patient care and achieve better outcomes. We have presented many examples in the case studies in this text to justify this hypothesis. The evidence in support increases every month. Improving quality and patient safety are two of the most important goals of healthcare organizations (organizational sustainability is a third). Efforts to achieve these goals are likely to be more effective and less expensive if they are informed by strong research evidence.

Endnotes

1. See, for example, Rousseau, D. M., and S. McCarthy, "Evidence-Based Management: Educating Managers from an Evidence-Based Perspective." *Academy of Management Learning and Education* 6 (1): 84–101; Pfeffer, J. and R. I. Sutton, *Hard Facts, Dangerous Half-Truths and Total Nonsense: Profiting from Evidence-Based Management.* Boston: Harvard Business School Press, 2006; and, in a related vein, Davenport, T. H., and J. G. Harris, *Competing on Analytics.* Boston: Harvard Business School Press, 2007.

2. We have tried and failed in trying to get funding for most of our management research projects.

References

Daft, R. L., and D. Marcic. 2006. *Understanding Management*, 5th edition. Mason, OH: Thompson-Southwestern.

Groopman, J. 2007. *How Doctors Think*. Boston: Houghton-Mifflin.

Kovner, A. R., and T. G. Rundall. 2006. "Evidence-Based Management Reconsidered." *Frontiers of Health Services Management* 22: 3–22.

METHODS FOR DEVELOPING ACTIONABLE EVIDENCE FOR CONSUMERS OF HEALTH SERVICES RESEARCH

John Hsu, Laura Arroyo, Ilana Graetz, Esther B. Neuwirth, Julie Schmittdiel, Thomas G. Rundall, Peter F. Martelli, Rodney McCurdy, Mark Gibson, and Pam Curtis

This excerpt from the Journal of Healthcare Management 52 (5): 335-41 *provides background, key points, guides, and checklists for the evidence-based decision-making process. Used with permission.*

Six Steps for Managers to Consider When Making a Well-informed Decision

Step 1: Framing the Question Behind the Decision
Background

The first step is to turn the management question into a research question, framing the issue in such a way that will increase the probability of locating useful research studies. This task requires more thought than one may first believe. Often, a very specific management question will have to be broadened to find relevant research, but overly broad, vague, or highly abstract research questions must be avoided.

Key Points
- Formulating your management decision question is the first step in finding relevant evidence.
- Care must be taken in the formulation of the management research question, making sure that the question is not overly broad or too narrow.

Guides and Checklists

When formulating your management decision question, consider the following five issues:

Issue 1: A well-defined question will explicitly state the intervention, outcome of interest, type of setting, timeframe, and population.

Issue 2: Each question should focus on a single information gap. A managerial decision, however, might involve several questions. If so, it is best to separate them into specific questions.

Issue 3: Questions should focus on objective criteria, rather than on value-based terms. For example, "which option is better?" is a value-laden decision; whereas, "which option is more likely to result in greater first year profit?" focuses on an objective outcome.

Issue 4: Some questions also should include information on the regulatory and reimbursement environment.

Issue 5: Identifying other important drivers of your decision also is critical. Examples of potentially important decision-making drivers include your market or political environment. Be sure to consider the decision from the viewpoint of other stakeholders.

Example

Imagine a manager wants to know whether to merge two hospitals:

What is the proposed change or intervention? In this example, the healthcare manager is interested in a merger between two healthcare organizations. Both organizations are hospitals in the same county, but different cities, i.e. this would be a horizontal merger between two hospitals.

What are the main outcomes of interest? Positive changes in these outcomes would represent a successful decision/implementation, whereas no or negative changes could represent poor implementation. In this example, the manager wants to know about the impact of the merger on pre-tax profits and quality of care.

What is the setting for the change? Think both about the internal organizational context as well as the broader market environment. Organizational context includes work climate and culture. For example, staff may resist the consolidation of managerial positions that have high institutional value; in other words, it may be difficult to turn two chairs of medicine into one. The market environment may include reimbursement, regulatory, or political concerns. In this example, both hospitals have capitated contracts with three health plans, which accounts for 80 percent of their admissions. Another example is that the manager is particularly concerned about integrating the leadership of the two hospitals or concerned that the two hospitals have different missions or orientations, e.g. one is for-profit and the other is not-for-profit.

What is the timeframe for the managerial changes and for the outcomes? In this example, the manager needs to present information on the merger implementation and outcomes after one year to her board of directors.

What are the relevant populations? In this example, the hospitals serve indigent, Medicare, and commercial insurance populations.

How does the intervention affect the outcomes of interest during the specified time period for the target population, within a specific environment? When the example information provided above is plugged into this template, the management decision question becomes:

How does a horizontal merger between two hospitals affect profitability and hospital quality outcomes during the first and subsequent years in a capitated environment with a substantial amount of charity care? With this question, you can now start to look for evidence related to your intervention. You also can focus your search on evidence that examines comparable outcomes within a similar context that you have now specified. Depending on the amount of available evidence, you may need to narrow or expand your definition of comparable outcomes, timeframes, environments, and populations.

The evidence that you find in the example does not tell you to merge the two hospitals or not, but can tell you what are likely effects on the two outcomes over the one-year and multi-year timeframes. If these are the two most important outcomes for deciding whether the option is "good" or "bad," then the evidence could indicate that mergers always yield positive outcome changes, always yield negative outcome changes, or produce some positive changes in one outcome and some negative changes in the other outcome for a given time period.

Step 2: Finding Sources of Information
Background

Evidence relevant to the management research question can be obtained from a wide array of sources. Colleagues, consultants, and known experts are frequent sources of colloquial evidence. Existing administrative and clinical data bases can be tapped for data. Pilot studies can be performed to collect data useful to a major decision.

Health organizations that have made significant investments in knowledge management may have libraries, trained librarians and webmasters, intranet information resources, or an in-house management decision-support system. The vast majority of managers will not have such resources, but will be limited to what they can find on the open Internet.

The Internet can be used to locate research articles and systematic reviews of multiple research studies. Two general approaches can be used to acquire research evidence via the open Internet:

• Searching websites that provide access to systematic reviews or meta-analyses (see Sidebar 7.1). For example, the Effective Practice and Organization of Care (EPOC) group within the Cochrane Library may provide insight. A research synthesis of a large number of primary research articles is especially useful to decision makers since the authors of the synthesis have already made an attempt to assess the quality of the evidence and to draw out the conclusions that are supported by the evidence.

- Searching bibliographic databases such as the National Library of Medicine Gateway and Google Scholar for published and unpublished primary studies of relevance to the research question.

Sidebar 7.1 Useful Websites

Many existing websites provide access to primary research studies or to summaries and syntheses of research that are useful to health services managers and policymakers. Some of the websites are listed here.

www.academyhealth.org
AcademyHealth

www.ahrq.gov/research
Agency for Healthcare Research and Quality research findings section

www.chsrf.ca
Canadian Health Services Research Foundation

www.depts.washington.edu/chmr
Center for Health Management Research

www.epoc.uottawa.ca
Cochrane Collaboration Effective Practice and Organization of Care Group

www.scholar.google.com
Google Scholar

www.ihi.org
Institute for Healthcare Improvement

www.gateway.nlm.nih.gov
National Library of Medicine Gateway

www.rwjf.org/publications/synthesis
The Robert Wood Johnson Foundation Synthesis Project

Key Points

Evidence to assist in decision-making can come from a variety of sources.

- Colloquial evidence can be obtained from the experience and judgment of colleagues, friends, customers, suppliers, and others. Information provided in organizational reports, trade journals, strategic planning sessions, offsite retreats, office meetings, and other settings may provide useful colloquial evidence.
- The focus of the Informed Decisions Toolbox is on finding research evidence.
- Research evidence can be generated within the organization, using administrative and clinical databases or by collecting new data using surveys or other techniques.
- Research evidence may also come from reports of studies conducted in other organizations, often published in academic journals or books.
- Research evidence on industry or environmental data and trends over time may be found in government reports, industry newswires, trade journals, conference proceedings, and other outlets.
- Internet websites sponsored by foundations, research centers, professional societies, publishers, and government agencies are particularly rich and accessible sources of colloquial and research evidence.
- Ability to search for and locate relevant research syntheses is an important competency (see Sidebar 7.2).

Librarians

Your organization may have a librarian that can help refine searches. If not, first consult a public library or local university library; it may be helpful to develop long-term relationships with these sources.

A list of medical and health services libraries is available through the University of Iowa: www.lib.uiowa.edu/hardin/hslibs.html. In extreme cases, a librarian at the National Library of Medicine may be able to help: www.nlm.nih.gov/contacts/contact.html.

Validating Organizations/External Standards

These resources include nationally recognized organizations such as the Agency for Healthcare Research and Quality (www.ahrq.gov), the Institute for Healthcare Improvement (www.ihi.org), or the Kaiser Family Foundation (www.kff.org). Many of these sites have white papers, position statements, or conference proceedings that can be downloaded.

Conferences and Other Professional Exchanges

Talking with colleagues can be a source of colloquial evidence. This evidence is generally not high quality, but can often be critical to finding further sources. Public administrators might consider contacting similar authorities in nearby states for guidance.

Knowledge Brokers, Consultants

Knowledge brokers often have special skills or resources, and can synthesize literature and offer advice. Brokers, including management consultants, may charge significant fees or require confidentiality agreements, which can exclude many from seeking this service.

Advocates, Vendors, and Advertisements

Advocates and vendors can have extremely detailed information on a given topic. However, the evidence they produce is generally biased in favor of their organizational mission. We feel that advocates and vendors sometimes fail to provide a full picture of available options. For this reason, we urge caution when dealing with these sources.

Databases and Internal Feedback

Some organizations have the capacity to collect, structure, and analyze data on organizational

---

Sidebar 7.2 Search Tips

- Simply enter key words from your management research question into the search field. For more advanced searches, the following tips will be helpful:
  - Start with a narrow topic using exact phrases and key words addressed in your management question.
  - When you find a hit, zoom out to explore citations, similar sources and authors, and links.
  - Use those resources to zoom in to find your answer.

Additional Tips

Phrase " "
   Using quotation marks limits the search to the phrase as written.
   Example: "health system merger"
Truncation *
   Using an asterisk will expand the search to all words beginning with those letters.
   Example: insur* will return insurance, insuring, insurer, and so on
Boolean AND, OR, NOT
   Using these words will combine, include, or exclude results.
   Example: health insurance NOT deductible

(continued)

Sidebar 7.2 (*continued*)

Note: Some engines, such as Google, do not recognize these terms. In these cases, use + or − instead.

  Example: health insurance
  −deductible

Limit search domain using site:.xyz

  Using the term "site:.xyz" will reduce all results to the domain .xyz. Available domains include .edu = academic, .gov = government, .org = organization, .com = commercial, .net = network, .mil = military, and so on. Example: health system merger site:.edu will reduce all results to academic websites.

processes. These data can directly provide an answer to particular operational questions, and offer insight for strategic decisions. Additionally, developing small-scale, short-term pilot studies for a management question acts as a test-run for a proposed intervention. Moderate research design and implementation skills are useful for this step, but even simple descriptive data analysis using basic mathematics can provide rich information.

Legal Resources

Laws and regulations in a given jurisdiction may have consequences for a decision. Legal information can be a valuable guide, but should always be checked with a counsel before being acted on. Good introductory resources can be found through the St. Louis University School of Law: http://law.slu.edu/healthlaw/research/links/index.html.

Steps 3–5: Evaluating the Evidence

Background

Not all evidence is of the same quality. Evidence that is of higher quality should be relied upon more than lower quality evidence. To assess the quality of a study, it is important to begin with an understanding of the study's design and the general strengths and weaknesses of that design. The following table provides brief comments on the strengths and weaknesses of various study designs that are commonly used in health services research.

Study Design	Comments
Meta-Analysis	The most rigorous way of synthesizing information. This approach, however, is limited by the quality of the supporting studies (i.e., a meta-analysis does not necessarily change the underlying validity of the studies).
Randomized Controlled Trial	The strongest study design for eliminating concerns about bias or confounding. The limitation of these

studies often is that the study sample is very homogeneous with numerous exclusions, thus limiting the applicability of any study results.

Quasi-Experimental Study	Can include many of the positive characteristics of the randomized controlled trial, but also a range of sub-designs. The most rigorous includes concurrent control groups and has multiple measurements over time, both before and after the intervention.
Prospective Cohort Study	Follows two or more groups prospectively.
Retrospective Cohort Study	Similar to the prospective cohort, but collects data afterwards. One major concern is that retrospectively collected data may not be the most desirable measurements or may be inaccurate (recall bias).
Case Control Study	Useful approach when data collection is expensive; common in epidemiological studies.
Uncontrolled Observational Study (no concurrent control)	Without a concurrent control group, the observed outcome changes may be because of other changes in the market (secular changes).
Qualitative Study	Useful for exploring new areas, identifying best practices, or understanding why a change has or has not occurred. These studies have small samples, which might not be similar to your organization. Other notable concerns include the transparency of the methods and potential subjectivity of the approach.

However, beyond the strengths and weaknesses of a study's design are many other issues that can affect the quality of the study and it findings. The following segment of the Informed Decisions Toolbox provides some Key Points to keep in mind when assessing evidence and some Guides and Checklists for making such an assessment.

Key Points

- Evidence must be accurate, applicable, actionable, and accessible.
- Inaccurate evidence can lead to bad decisions.
- Inapplicable evidence may have little value for your decision.
- Evidence that is not easily actionable will be difficult to use or implement.
- Evidence that is difficult to access can be prohibitively costly to obtain (time or money).
- Evaluating evidence is a critical step in the decision-making process.

Four A's of Useful Evidence

Useful evidence is Accurate, Applicable, Actionable, and Accessible.

Accurate
- Establishes causal relationship, not "expert opinion"
- Provides a complete, balanced viewpoint
- Provides information on relevant statistical properties, without necessarily eliminating data based on arbitrary standards of precision
- Provides information on limitations
- Is a credible source—unbiased support (funding) and implementation
- Uses a transparent process—how data are collected and findings follow from data
- Is based on observational studies and tacit information

Applicable
- Research is relevant to the decision maker's question
- Research states in which situations it is applicable
- Information is applicable to the decision maker's organization and environment

Actionable
- Fits into the time frame of the original decision
- Includes information on what needs to be done
- Provides information on a complete set of implications, including costs, overall importance, and values
- Identifies best practices
- Includes measurable quality indicators
- Portrays expected vs. actual outcomes
- Should evaluate usefulness of technology
- Considers context, including other available information, e.g., includes tacit information

Accessible
- Easy to obtain—at our fingertips
- Presentation framing consistent with decision-maker needs

Step 3: Assessing the Accuracy of Information
Questions for Quantitative Evidence: Do I Have Accurate Information?

Are the research findings valid?
- ❑ Does the study provide interpretable information about its sample definition and size, including the specific inclusion and exclusion criteria?
- ❑ Do these criteria exclude any groups or subjects that would make the findings less valid or interpretable?
- ❑ What was the study design? Is it a strong design (see previous table—Study Design)?
- ❑ Does the study provide interpretable information about its context and setting?
- ❑ Do the study results indicate that the intervention led to the outcome changes (i.e. a causal relationship)?
- ❑ Are the methods for collecting data transparent and clearly presented?
- ❑ Are the measurements reliable and valid? Is there a gold standard for these measurements?
- ❑ Is the association between the findings and the results (data) clearly defined?
- ❑ Does the study control for other concurrent changes that could influence the outcome (concurrent control groups and adjustment for potential confounders)?

Does the evidence provide a complete and balanced viewpoint, "The Good, Bad, and Ugly?"
- ❑ Does the study address all of the important options and outcomes?
- ❑ Does the study list its limitations?
- ❑ Does the study discuss its findings within the context of other previous studies, tacit knowledge, or original expectations?

Was the analysis appropriate (correct use of statistics)?
- ❑ Does the study state how it performed its analyses?
- ❑ Does the study examine whether the assumptions behind the analytic methods were correct?
- ❑ Does the study perform sensitivity analyses to assess the impact of its assumptions?
- ❑ Does the study discuss alternative explanations that it was not able to measure (unmeasured confounders)?
- ❑ What were the best estimates of the intervention effects? The point estimates generally arc the best assessment of the "true" effect.

❏ How precise were the results? The p-values or confidence intervals provide information about whether these estimates of the intervention effect could have been due to chance. Often managerial studies will have limited power (i.e., less precision of its estimates) to detect changes. In this situation, the point estimates remain the best assessment of the "true effect." Whether the level of precision is adequate for your decision requires you to weight the available evidence. In other words, "statistically insignificant" results could still be useful for your decision. Conversely, "statistically significant" results do not mean that these are operationally meaningful, especially if the intervention appears to have a small effect (operationally insignificant effect size).

Is the source credible?
❏ Who conducted the study? Does the study list any potential conflicts of interest for the investigators?
❏ Who paid for the study?
❏ Did any group other than the investigators have the ability to censor or modify the study results?
❏ Did any group other than the investigators have the ability to censor or modify the study interpretation (conclusions)?

Questions for Qualitative Evidence: Do I Have Accurate Information?

Understanding the Context:
❏ Is the context of the study adequately described?
❏ Are the research aims/objectives/questions clearly defined and focused?
❏ Are the methods used appropriate to the research question?

Understanding the Sample Selection:
❏ How does the study select its sample? Qualitative studies often use a small, "purposeful" sample. Is this approach clearly presented?
❏ Is the study sample sufficient to understand the study context and population?
❏ Was the sampling predetermined or did it evolve as the fieldwork progressed?
❏ Who was selected and why (consider gender, age, ethnicity, marital status, professional role)?
❏ Is it clear why some participants were not selected?

Understanding the Data Collection Process:
❏ How were data collected?
❏ Were data collection tools pilot tested?
❏ How were the data recorded and why (tape recorded, notes, etc.)?

Assessing the Analysis:
- ❏ Who conducted the research and how were they selected?
- ❏ Were the researcher's skills and motives discussed?
- ❏ Is it clear how the researcher processed the raw data to arrive at the stated results?
- ❏ Were the categories and themes identified in advance, or derived from the data?
- ❏ Are all data taken into account in the analysis?
- ❏ Are responses/experiences compared or contrasted across different groups/individuals/study sites?
- ❏ Did more than one person identify themes and code transcripts?
- ❏ Did the researcher check to see whether the coding approach was consistent across multiple coders (reliability of the coding)?

Assessing the Validity of Findings:
- ❏ How did the researcher assess whether the methods were valid?
- ❏ Does the study look for examples that do not fit its findings (counter-factual examples)?
- ❏ Did the researcher review the study's findings with the original subjects to assess the accuracy of the interpretation?
- ❏ Does the study present information on the actual data?
- ❏ Does the study provide a credible link between the presented data and the stated results?
- ❏ Does the study provide a credible link between the stated results and the main conclusions?

Step 4: Assessing the Applicability of Information
Questions for Applicable Evidence
- ❏ Is the study sample comparable to your population?
- ❏ Is the study setting comparable to your organization?
- ❏ Is the study context comparable to your organization's environment and market?
- ❏ Is the study intervention comparable to your intervention?
- ❏ Are the study outcomes comparable to your outcomes of interest?
- ❏ Is the timeframe of the study outcomes comparable to the time frame of your outcomes of interest?
- ❏ Does the study indicate when the findings are applicable?

Step 5: Assessing the Actionability of Information
Questions for Actionable Evidence

Is there information on what needs to be done?
- ❏ Are there examples of best practices?

❏ Is there information on a complete set of relevant implications, including costs, user perceptions, and impact on revenue?

Is there information on how to do it?
❏ Is there a discussion of implementation process?
❏ Is there information on who needs to do it?

Is there information on how to monitor whether it is working?
❏ Are there measurable indicators?
❏ Are these indicators feasible for your organization?

Step 6: Determining if the Information is Adequate

Given your organization's needs, values, and context, the evidence may indicate (1) that one option is clearly desirable or undesirable; (2) that more than one option may be reasonable depending on how the organization values the likely effects, i.e., there are tradeoffs; or (3) that none of the options have adequate information for the decision.

If one option is clearly desirable (or undesirable), i.e. it is the dominant strategy given your organization's needs, values, and context, then you have a definitive answer. This situation may occur infrequently.

If more than one option is reasonable, but each has different strengths and weaknesses, then you may have a series of tradeoffs. With these specified options and delineated tradeoffs, you can now start your decision-making process.

If none of the options are reasonable or have adequate information, then you need to decide how important collecting this information would be.

Often, the available research evidence is most useful in specifying and informing the tradeoffs associated with the decision option. This approach can help improve the organization's understanding of the underlying question/problem, encourage communication between stakeholders, help managers develop new solutions, or anticipate future effects (enlightenment process).

Given multiple reasonable options requiring tradeoffs, a deliberative process is one useful approach.

Questions for Using Evidence—Do I Have Adequate Information for This Decision?

General
❏ What are your decision options?
❏ Do I have a complete list of options?
❏ What does the available credible evidence indicate about each of your decision options?

❏ Is there a dominant option? More than one option involving trade-offs? Inadequate information?

Single Option—Dominant Strategies
❏ Is there a single decision option that dominates all of your outcome criteria?
❏ Is this option always better than the other options with respect to your criteria?
❏ Is this option always worse than the other options with respect to your criteria?

Multiple Options—Tradeoffs
❏ Is there more than one viable option after reviewing the available credible evidence?
❏ Do these options have different strengths and weakness with respect to your outcomes and decision-making criteria?
❏ What are the tradeoffs associated with each option?

Uncertain Options—Inadequate Information
❏ Is there more than one remaining decision option after reviewing the available credible evidence?
❏ Do these options have uncertain strengths and weaknesses with respect to your outcomes and decision-making criteria?

LOOK IT UP

Sara Mody, with an introduction by Anthony R. Kovner

Introduction

Sara Mody, a first-year graduate student at NYU/Wagner, wrote the following piece to help graduate students in healthcare management follow an evidence-based approach. I asked her to imagine she was an administrative fellow of a large health system assigned to research "hospital governance"—a topic with which I was already familiar. My secondary motive was to validate that I had a good handle on the information surrounding the subject.

What might a CEO do after reading the one-page presentation on hospital governance that Sara prepared (presented at the end of this chapter)? The CEO might do nothing, or she might ask Sara to go back and find additional evidence in the literature or from other sources on the issues.

As an example of how a CEO might push an issue further, let's focus on a topic the memo raises: the value of setting measurable objectives. Let's assume the hospital board does not set measurable objectives, share them with key stakeholders, report quarterly on attainment of objectives, or regularly change objectives or strategies as circumstances change. This notion is mine, not Sara's, although she does provide evidence supporting the value of measureable objectives, obtained from literature on effective hospital boards:

- The board monitors the financial health of the organization. It establishes financial objectives, ensures financial planning, requires strong financial performance, and invests prudently.
- The board handles executive human resource issues, including recruitment, the establishment of performance expectations, salary determination, and termination.
- The board measures performance (including its own performance), evaluating both financial and quality indicators.

If the CEO were to use this information to begin a consideration of governance practices, Sara's concise presentation would be considered successful.

Although not part of the assignment, the memo does not demonstrate how the CEO, and presumably the board chair, would implement a change in board culture. This process is discussed extensively in research literature and documented experience. Cultural change is a difficult and risky undertaking that the CEO and board chair may not wish to pursue. If they do pursue it, they should do everything they can to execute the task successfully.

Anthony R. Kovner

Look It Up

As an administrative fellow, I am asked to participate in a variety of projects and data collection activities around the hospital. Most recently, I was asked to evaluate our hospital board's performance. Administration knew the board was not operating to its potential and asked me to find out what we could do to make the board more effective.

Our board is made up of intelligent self-starters who generally pay little attention to hospital affairs outside of board meetings. Many of its elderly members received board appointment because they were friends of an effective chair several years ago, while others were invited to join the board because they were substantial donors to the hospital. Telling them they were doing a bad job without furnishing evidence would have made them immediately defensive. Moreover, they were not necessarily doing a bad job; rather, they were doing a job different from the one administration expected. Specifically, the board and administration disagreed on what the board was doing and how it was using its role.

Using the evidence-based approach to address this question allows a hospital's administration to take opinions and feelings out of the equation. If the administration's position is that it needs to ask more of the board, it will need evidence to support it. More important, the administration must convince the board of the need for change. Evidence that high-performing boards have a positive effect on their organizations' overall performance will help the board understand the benefits of change. Evidence also will enable the hospital and board to establish measurable, shared objectives, without which there is no accountability. Ultimately, the board should understand the issue is not someone "thinking" the board is ineffective; instead, both the board and administration must know the board could be more effective.

Given the number of other projects I was working on, I could not dedicate more than 40 hours to finding an answer to this situation. I planned to spend about half a day framing the question and discussing the final research question(s) with the CEO, one day researching, two days evaluating the research, and one day organizing the applicable research for further use.

Day One: Framing the Question

Before I could begin my research, I needed to figure out what the hospital administration meant by "effective." If the board had the wrong people (e.g., they didn't have the desired expertise, conflicts of interest existed, they were poor leaders) or the wrong structure (e.g., there were too many or too few members, the meeting format didn't work, the hospital leadership and board didn't communicate well), it would no doubt be ineffective. Even with the ideal people and correct structure, the board could still be considered ineffective if members did not have a clear understanding of their role. Before addressing people or structure, I needed to define board objectives. People and structure, although important, can be addressed in the implementation phase of the change initiative.

While meeting to discuss my definition of the research question, the CEO and I added another element: finding evidence to support measurement of board performance. This addition raised two questions: Is good board performance a criterion for effective operation? If so, what should an organization use to measure board performance?

We also decided that, in the interest of time, we should use only the most recent research. We determined that articles published between 2000 and 2007 would suffice. Useful older articles would be cited in the more recent articles.

Day Two: Finding Sources of Information

I started my search with Google Scholar. I entered the search criteria "hospital + board + composition," which returned 40,800 hits. The search criteria "hospital + board + governance + best practice" returned 19,200 hits. My final search of "hospital + board + governance" returned 23,500 hits. Unfortunately, while I had thousands of possible articles, none of the search criteria quickly led me to what I needed.

Search Tips: Google Scholar works well—sometimes. I found that the search engine usually will give you what you need in the first 20 articles returned. Google Scholar's "Advanced Scholar Search" limits the number of relevant hits in many cases, since you can specify publication, date, and subject area in addition to the normal key word and phrase specifics.

I then searched another large database of journal articles, PubMed.

Search Tips: If you are unsure which academic journals publish articles on the topic you are interested in, a database of journals can guide you. Again, you can sort the results by date of publication. When you select an article or abstract, PubMed has a useful "Related Links" feature that displays a listing of similar articles.

I searched for "hospital board" (1,036 hits) and "board relations" (1,843 hits).

The first search proved to be the most useful. Since I was interested in only the most recent academic research, I sorted the hits by publication date. A recent article in the *Journal of Healthcare Management* titled "Hospital Governing Boards: A Study of Their Effectiveness in Relation to Organizational Performance" was tenth in my list of search results. I could not have asked for a more relevant article. The Related Links feature offered 103 similar articles, of which 34 were published after 2000. From title alone I determined that some were not relevant, but in the end, I had 12 articles to review more closely—a much more manageable number than the original 40,800.

Now that I had found the potentially relevant journal articles, I looked to see what the major research organizations might offer. I browsed the websites of the Center for Health Management Research, the Advisory Board Company, the Canadian Health Services Research Foundation (CHSRF), the Governance Institute, and the Health Research and Educational Trust. CHSRF's site returned 287 hits when I searched for "governance"; however, none of the articles appeared applicable. The Advisory Board's site had some potentially relevant articles, but membership was required to access the most promising ones. The Governance Institute and Health Research and Educational Trust sites were most helpful; both supplied some useful sources.

Days Three and Four: Evaluating the Evidence

Pfeffer and Sutton (2006) could not have put it better—when looking at research, you need to determine the difference between "hard facts, dangerous half-truths, and total nonsense." As I began reviewing the articles, I noticed that I had a mix of empirical studies, qualitative studies, and anecdotal advice. I had to determine what reliable evidence looked like. The best way to explain the difference between "good" evidence and "better" evidence is to walk through an evaluation of two journal articles. Both articles came from trustworthy healthcare journals, which shows you cannot rely on journal name alone to provide solid, actionable evidence.

The Good Evidence

In spring 2005, a journal published by the American College of Healthcare Executives, *Frontiers of Health Services Management*, ran an article by E. George Middleton, Jr. (2005), titled "Priority Issues for Hospital Boards." The author is a board member of a successful hospital system in Virginia. The title of the paper suggested it would contain exactly what I needed to know. At first glance, the article appeared reliable and relevant.

Middleton explains the most important functions for a hospital board and provides recommendations for implementation. He identifies issues such as member qualification, board structure, quality, and compliance as key focus areas, supporting each topic with compelling arguments. While there is nothing inherently wrong with the priorities he listed, there is also nothing obviously right about them, either. The author did not perform quantitative or qualitative research. In fact, Middleton supports his suggestions with only one reference in the entire ten-page article. Instead, he bases his comments on personal experience, insights, and opinions. As much value as they may have, without supporting evidence, I was reluctant to put much stock in what might be "dangerous half-truths."

The Better Evidence

As mentioned earlier, the *Journal of Healthcare Management* had published an article regarding a board's impact on hospital effectiveness. The article begins with a summary of the changes governing boards have experienced in recent years. After reviewing the current literature, the author, Kathryn J. McDonagh (2006), concludes that two questions remain unanswered: Do boards really make a difference? How can boards improve hospital performance?

To pursue these two inquiries, the author framed the following research questions: Are the six competency factors in the BSAQ (Board Self-Assessment Questionnaire) tool widely used in nonprofit organizations similar to those used in nonprofit hospitals? Do better-performing boards result in better-performing hospitals? (The BSAQ has been tested extensively and is widely considered reliable. It measures board performance along six dimensions: contextual, educational, interpersonal, analytical, political, and strategic.) McDonagh collected data using convenience sampling over a four-month period. One hundred fifty-one CEOs and other organizational leaders from 64 hospitals around the country responded, yielding a 13 percent response rate. McDonagh based hospital performance on Solucient's 100 Top Hospitals program, a ranking system frequently used in other studies.

The author describes in detail the statistical techniques she used to evaluate the data. Factor analyses supported the common thought that successful boards work as cohesive teams. Single-factor findings drew attention away from the usual "keys" to board success—size, composition, and term limits—and brought it toward the idea of boards as social systems.

Most important, the research showed that high-performing boards were more likely to be leading better-performing hospitals, particularly in terms of profitability and expense management. Higher-performing boards also showed lower BSAQ scores on the "political" dimension, which means they focus on relationships with key stakeholders, without letting politics get in the way. The article concludes with the author's recommendations for applying the findings. The paper clearly displays findings and statistical correlations in easy-to-understand tables. A strong sample, reliable statistical analysis, applicable findings, and clear presentation led me to consider the results of this study "hard facts."

The Evidence: Bottom Line

The caution in relying heavily on Middleton's article lies in the lack of support for his assertions. While his recommendations may be correct, they may appear less convincing to board members, who might believe they could just as easily find a paper written by someone with opposing views. Evidence should support legitimate initiatives, not lead the group into a battle of opinions.

I found McDonagh's strong evidence noteworthy, but I found the general recommendations for board objectives lacking. For instance, the evidence supports the need for boards' building strong relationships with key stakeholders, but does not clearly define who should be included in the "key stakeholder" mix. More in-depth research could be performed on each of the general recommendations to clarify them.

While a continued literature review would have been useful, I decided to try to access additional information through other sources. For example, the hospital executives could get input from their contacts on high-performing boards in noncompeting areas or other hospitals within the system. Or the hospital could establish a partnership with a local university to obtain the advice of an academic expert on board relations. Literature provides quick access to information, but if time allows, personal interviews and informal conversations may provide a deeper understanding.

Day Five: Organizing and Presenting Findings

Ultimately, I used seven articles from my PubMed search, one article from the Governance Institute, and one from the Health Research and Educational Trust. After picking my final sources, I needed to find an easy way to present the information to the CEO. Given the value of her time, I put together a one-page guide to the research. The guide walked the reader through common board perceptions, two models of governance, board objectives, and key takeaways.

In addition, I created an annotated bibliography that grouped my sources into two categories—empirical studies and qualitative studies (see the Appendix to this chapter). I intended for the bibliography to lead the administrators and board members through the research methodology and key findings for each source cited in the guide.

During my presentation to the CEO, I walked her through the one-page brief and recommended the following:

- First, I emphasized the importance of identifying a board champion to help lead the change initiative. The board champion would give key stakeholders a voice and involve them in the change process.
- I recommended contracting an outside consultant to facilitate the process. The consultant could help guide the board and administration and ensure

that the new structure aligned with the hospital's mission and vision.
- The hospital would also need an easy way to monitor the board's performance once goals were established. I proposed the services of a nonprofit organization called BoardSource (www.boardsource.org), which has a multitude of electronic tools for this purpose.
- Last, I suggested recruiting board members with a history of participation in successful boards.

Conclusion

Upon reflection, a few other important points come to mind. Setting the research question remains a crucial step to producing an end product that people will use. I have a tendency to get ahead of myself and jump right into the research process. I didn't fully understand the value of discussing the question with the CEO until later, when I started digging through hundreds of articles. The question kept me focused on the end purpose of my research.

This assignment also helped me realize the importance of setting research standards. When is research too old to be relevant? Can the research question be sufficiently answered on qualitative evidence alone? What qualifies as good evidence? Deciding beforehand what I thought the end users would consider reliable evidence helped me manage the research process, and I quickly learned to differentiate between good advice and untested recommendations.

Finally, I concluded that it was not important to produce a lengthy document to demonstrate how much research I had done. Instead, I chose quality over quantity. A handful of reliable sources will prove more useful than a plethora of opinions and hearsay.

Appendix

Do Effective Boards Lead to Better Performing Hospitals? Yes.

Editor's Note: This appendix is an example of the research one could put together for an administrator. This shows research does not have to be an overwhelming amount of information. Presenting information succinctly makes the research manageable and actionable.

Common Board Views

Surveyed board members did not believe governing board performance strongly correlated to hospital financial performance. In order from most to least important, they ranked market conditions, clinical expertise, and CEO performance above board performance (McDonagh 2006).

Types of Governance Models

- **Philanthropic Characteristics:** emphasis on community participation, due process, and stewardship
- **Corporate Characteristics:** emphasis on strategy development, risk taking, and competitive positioning
- **Research** (Alexander and Lee 2006):
  - Philanthropic-style boards are more likely to close their hospitals under conditions of low organizational performance
  - Hospitals governed by corporate-style boards are more likely to be more efficient, have higher admissions, and possess a greater market share

Philanthropic	Corporate
Large board size, wide range of backgrounds	Small board size; narrow, more focused backgrounds
Small number of inside directors	Large number of inside directors
Little management participation	Active management participation
No formal management accountability to board	Direct management accountability to board
No limit for consecutive terms for board members	Limit to consecutive terms for board members
No compensation for board service	Compensation for board service
Emphasis on asset preservation	Emphasis on strategic activity

SOURCE: Alexander and Lee (2006).

Board Objectives

- Oversee internal operations—manage relationships; monitor quality, safety, and clinical outcomes; maintain physician relationships (Margolin et al. 2005; National Quality Forum 2005; Pointer and Ewell 1995; Foster 2006).
- Build relationships with external stakeholders. This role includes fundraising obligations assumed by 35 percent of boards surveyed (Margolin et al. 2005).
- Help shape the future of the organization through strategic planning and crafting the mission and vision. Fifty-nine percent of hospitals

have strategic planning committees (Margolin et al. 2005; Pointer and Ewell 1995).

- Monitor the financial health of the organization—establish financial objectives, ensure financial planning, require strong financial performance, invest prudently (Pointer and Ewell 1995).
- Evaluate executive performance—including recruiting, setting performance expectations, determining compensation, and termination (Pointer and Ewell 1995, Foster 2006).

Measurement

- Sixty-five percent of boards measure their own performance against established standards. Of this group, 74 percent evaluate the total board; 86 percent perform an annual assessment. (Margolin et al. 2005).
- Financial data are used by 92 percent of boards as a measurement of performance (Margolin et al. 2005).
- Performance indicators vary based on board model (Alexander and Lee 2006).

What Really Matters?

- Acting as a "collaborative, community oriented, and socially dynamic network of leaders dedicated to a unified purpose" (McDonagh 2006; Sonnenfeld 2002)
- Measuring performance—evaluating both financial and quality indicators (National Quality Forum 2005; Pointer and Ewell 1995)
- Creating "a virtuous cycle of respect, trust, and candor" (Sonnenfeld 2002)
- Welcoming a "dialogue, debate, and constructive dissent" (Productive boards are interactive and proactive, and make an effort to lessen impact of politics.) (Prybil 2006; Sonnenfeld 2002; McDonagh 2006)
- Supporting a "fluid portfolio of roles" (Members should challenge their own roles and assumptions [Sonnenfeld 2002]. Boards play an integral part in policy formation, decision making, and oversight [Pointer and Ewell 1995].)
- Requiring individual accountability (Assign individual responsibilities.) (Sonnenfeld 2002)

Keys for Successful Change

Have a board champion; seek an experienced, external facilitator; allow key stakeholders to have an influential role; align governance structure with mission and vision; recruit board members with a history of participating in successful boards (Knecht and Kazemek 2001).

References

Alexander, J. A., and S. D. Lee. 2006. "Does Governance Matter? Board Configuration and Performance in Not-for-Profit Hospitals." *Milbank Quarterly* 84 (4): 733–58.

Foster, D. 2006. *Correlations Between Board Quality Oversight and Successful Hospital Performance.* San Diego: The Governance Institute.

Knecht, P. R., and E. A. Kazemek. 2001. "Whose Job Is It Anyway?" *Trustee* 54 (8): 16–20.

McDonagh, K. 2006. "Hospital Governing Boards: A Study of Their Effectiveness in Relation to Organizational Performance." *Journal of Healthcare Management* 51: 377–89.

Margolin, F. S., S. Hawkins, J. A. Alexander, and L. Prybil. 2005. *Hospital Governance: Initial Summary Report of 2005 Survey of CEOs and Board Chairs.* Chicago: Health Research and Educational Trust.

Middleton, E. G., Jr. 2005. "Priority Issues for Hospital Boards." *Frontiers of Health Services Management* 21: 13–24.

National Quality Forum. 2005. "Hospital Governing Boards and Quality of Care: A Call to Responsibility." *Trustee* 58 (3): 15–18.

Pfeffer, J., and R. Sutton. 2006. *Hard Facts, Dangerous Half-Truths and Total Nonsense: Profiting from Evidence-Based Management.* Boston: Harvard Business School Press.

Pointer, D. D., and C. M. Ewell. 1995. "Really Governing: What Type of Work Should Boards Be Doing?" *Hospital & Health Services Administration* 40 (3): 315–31.

Prybil, L. D. 2006. "Size, Composition, and Culture of High-Performing Hospital Boards." *American Journal of Medical Quality* 21 (224): 224–29.

Sonnenfeld, J. A. 2002. "What Makes Great Boards Great?" *Harvard Business Review* 80 (9): 106–13, 126.

CASE STUDIES OF MANAGEMENT INTERVENTIONS USING AN EVIDENCE-BASED MANAGEMENT APPROACH

INTRODUCTION TO THE CASE STUDIES

Anthony R. Kovner, Richard D'Aquila, and David J. Fine, with the assistance of Sara Mody

The ten case studies that follow describe management interventions that used some approximation of the evidence-based approach. These interventions were carried out and evaluated by the writers, all of whom are managers and researchers known to the co-authors. In some instances, EB management techniques were used from the outset of a project, and in some, the EB management framework was applied retrospectively to initiatives already underway or completed. Some of the cases explicitly follow the steps of the EB management process, whereas others followed only some of the steps, or failed to report some steps. Yet all of the cases illustrate how to bring the underlying principles of EB management to bear on a management challenge.

We believe discussion and analysis of these cases will encourage those who study and practice healthcare management to use a more evidence-based approach in responding to management challenges. As Berwick (2007) puts it, "our world is a world of true complexity, strong social influences, tight dependence on local context, a world less of proof than of navigation, less of final conclusions than of continual learning, a world not of certainty about the past but of uncertain predictions and tentative plans about the future."

A wide range of important and timely management challenges is covered in these cases: disaster planning, leadership development, chronic care management, pain management, the improvement of health status of underserved children, the business case for a hospital palliative care unit, CEO evaluation, inpatient bed planning, and operating room scheduling.

None of the writers was able to satisfactorily analyze the costs and benefits of using EB management techniques. We do not suggest that these experiences can be generalized to other managers and management interventions, with respect to the amount of effort involved in the EB management process or its outcomes. Yet all the writers appear convinced that their efforts have led to improvements in their organizations, which are some of the nation's most complex healthcare enterprises.

This introduction provides a quick look at each case, enabling readers to focus on certain topics or themes. The most common characteristic of these case studies is that the managers, in considering problem-solving interventions, have usually taken great care to properly frame their management challenges and researchable problems. They then obtain and evaluate the evidence, adapt the evidence to the situation, and assess actionability before implementing the intervention. A common shortcoming in many of the cases is the heavy reliance on internal evidence, rather than on the literature and benchmarking with other organizations. Most of the writers also are silent as to the nature of the deliberative process and any retrospective look they took to see whether the promised benefits and predicted costs actually materialized.

The following text summarizes, for each case, the problem addressed, the research question, commentary, and the perceived benefits of an EB management approach.

Leadership Development at the Saint Boniface Healthcare System (page 121)

Problem: The pre-intervention leadership development program at Saint Boniface Healthcare System (SBHCS) was not improving succession readiness or fostering internal promotions.

Research question: What competencies among SBHCS senior decision makers would prepare them for advancement, and what competency-enhancing mechanisms produce the best leadership succession readiness outcomes?

Comment: The setting of this case, written by Philip DiSalvio, is a large health system that comprises seven acute care hospitals and other facilities and, with more than 22,000 employees and 4,750 physicians, is the second largest employer in its state. The management question was first phrased as: How do we conduct leadership development programs? The research question implies that producing the best outcomes in the most cost-effective way is the goal of the programs. To gather evidence, top management had to specify assumptions regarding the desired succession readiness level, the factors that contribute to reaching that level, and the costs and benefits of achieving it.

Had managers gathered evidence related to the benefits and costs of the leadership program that did not involve succession readiness, they might have been able to determine whether succession readiness or management effectiveness was the real issue. Research suggests they should expect these benefits from a management leadership development program: perception of a positive benefit among employees wishing to become managers or better managers; increased perception among senior managers of the importance of leadership development; and an increased focus by managers on factors that facilitate such development (for example, focus on empowering those who report directly to them). The leadership development program also draws attention to the increased priority on making changes to SBHCS's performance appraisal system, which will affect implementation of the evidence-based solution.

Results of EB management: SBHCS is in the process of changing the format and delivery of its Leadership Institute, so it is too early to report end results. However, EB management did bring about the use of tools that provide quantifiable feedback and performance metrics. SBHCS now has the ability to easily track outcomes like job movement, organizational advancement, and readiness in one place, through the Employment Initiative Dashboard Report.

Forming a Corporate University: More of the Same, or Something New? (page 137)

Problem: Training and development efforts at Best Health System were not equipping employees with the skills to move up in the organization, and those who did move up did not appear to be adequately prepared for their new roles. The system constantly had to recruit outside the organization for high-quality management candidates.

Research question: Would developing a corporate university at Best Health solve the system's human resources and organizational development issues?

Comment: This case, written by Ann McAlearney, explores a research question similar to that in the first case study: Should this large midwestern hospital start an in-house management development program? Alternative research questions could have been framed as: What is the current level of management skills and experience? What is the *desired* level, and how can the hospital's top management achieve it at acceptable costs? Top management then had to determine how managers are and should be selected and evaluated, how learning and improved effectiveness should be measured, and who should be accountable for program results among the managers being trained, their supervisors, and the department of human resources.

The author superbly reviewed research evidence on corporate universities and other approaches to management development. Her fine work reflects her previous experience conducting externally funded major exploratory research projects on this topic, in which she had reviewed the print and online literature and conducted a wide-ranging series of interviews with managers. This case illustrates how deep knowledge of a subject can focus the evidence-based approach.

Results of EB management: The EB management process enabled development of four evidence-supported options to address the system's issues. The evidence then helped guide the selection of one among them. Most important, strong evidence helped the system move to something unfamiliar and unprecedented—in other words, creating a solid business case made a critical strategy move less risky.

Transforming CEO Evaluation in a Multi-Unit Healthcare Organization (page 153)

Problem: The CEO evaluation process was informal, qualitative, and unstructured.

Research question: Can the CEO evaluation process be redesigned to provide a solid platform for accountability?

Comment: This case, written by Lawrence Prybil and colleagues, describes the transformation of a lackluster CEO evaluation process to one based on reasonable goals, performance criteria, and actionable feedback. A different research question could have been asked: To what extent can demonstrable improvements in institutional performance such as quality, financial performance, and patient satisfaction be correlated with improved accountability for executive performance? The case is silent as to the source of the performance goals established, the evidence supporting the selection of data to measure progress toward the goals, and the evidence used to determine the driving principles of the new evaluation process. Nor does it explore how CEO performance goals and targets mesh with those for hospital-wide performance.

The case presents an intuitive framework for holding senior management responsible for measurable targets. These principles should be applied to all levels of management and to the organization's workforce at large. Holding an entire organization to reasonable, measurable targets related to patient quality, customer satisfaction, financial performance, and regulatory readiness—then linking incentive compensation to these targets—provides the framework for extraordinary performance and alignment across all levels of the organization.

Results of EB management: The new process fosters accountability and is more transparent and participative. It allows each board member to be actively involved in setting objectives, rating performance against targets, and providing fair and actionable feedback directly to the CEO.

Improving Pain Management in Long-Term Care (page 161)

Problem: Village Care of New York initiated a quality improvement program focusing on pain management to better serve its geriatric and HIV/AIDS patients, for whom pain management is a principal issue.

Research question: Can an evidence-based pain management initiative using a quality improvement approach improve bedside care across 14 diverse programs?

Comment: Arthur Webb and Ellen Flaherty apply an evidence-based approach to pain management initiatives in the multiple programs and sites operated by Village Care of New York. The process presented in the case underscores their real-world struggle to establish a literature-based model (the Institute of Medicine's ideal of safe, efficient, patient centered, timely, effective, equitable care) to promote evidence-based changes in the treatment of chronic pain. The pre- and post-intervention metrics are not available in the case.

The program's success was based on achievement of a series of performance management quality goals. Leadership training for approximately 120 middle managers and an integrated team approach were the greatest contributors. Opportunities for future uses of EB management at Village Care include the authors' challenge to gain manager confidence and trust in research evidence that is not well understood at the organization's operational level.

Given that top management appears committed to the use of empirical research to help the organization become results driven and person centered, consideration should be given to allocating as little as one-quarter of 1 percent of its human capital and a similar slice of its cash flow to a small but dedicated team of "transformationalists" who can educate and guide internal champions in this and other projects.

Results of EB management: The case demonstrates how to use EB management with evidence-based medicine. EB management led Village Care to the idea of performance measurement as a means of quality improvement, while evidence-based medicine helped it determine necessary changes to the pain management program.

The Business Case for a Hospital Palliative Care Unit: Justifying Its Continued Existence (page 171)

Problem: An external consulting firm deemed the hospital's palliative care unit (PCU) unprofitable and strongly recommended that it be closed as one step toward maintaining the hospital's financial stability.

Research question: Does the evidence support the continued existence of the PCU from a patient outcome and financial point of view?

Comment: Kenneth White and J. Brian Cassel discuss the successful use of an EB management approach to prevent a hospital PCU's closure as part of an apparently urgent, hospital-wide cost-reduction program. Their study design depended exclusively on internal financial data, an often weak link in the U.S. hospital sector. (These data were the same the outside consulting group used in assessing all programs under review at the medical center.)

The case demonstrated that a distinct, 11-bed PCU staffed by a multidisciplinary care team saved the hospital approximately $3 million over three years and was even profitable for a subset of patients. The authors' research findings also indicated other strategies the hospital could use to cover the costs of care.

Of particular note in this case study is a circumstance in which apparently accurate data nonetheless can result in flawed recommendations. The EB management approach described in the case revealed the fallacy of the consultants' analytic methodology.

Results of EB management: EB management enabled the hospital to keep the PCU open, which allowed it to continue to provide much-needed, high-quality care. A thorough financial analysis also helped the unit identify the real issues and create a focused action plan to deal with them.

Using Evidence in Integrated Chronic Care Management (page 181)

Problem: Depression affects a large number of Americans. The pain, suffering, and cost can be reduced through proper treatment. However, most patients, if they do seek treatment, seek care from a primary care physician, not a mental health specialist. Primary care physicians do not have the clinical expertise, information systems, workflow techniques, or other evidence-based tools to effectively treat this chronic illness.

Research question: Can depression care be delivered to more individuals at their points of entry into the healthcare system? If so, how?

Comment: Kyle Grazier presents an intriguing study with a case-control experimental design seeking to inform the treatment of depression by primary care physicians. The research question differs fundamentally from typical management problem solving but embraces the broad spirit of EB management. A 1995 *British Medical Journal* report of a randomized controlled trial of the treatment of major depression using amitriptyline prescribed in the primary care setting provides the clinical foundation for the case. Published literature related to the bundle of services that would be implemented in the "case" practices but not in the "control" practices provided information about the need to identify clinical champions for the proposed intervention, the need for shared medical and mental health information, the education needed by providers and staff, and the importance of readily available specialist consultation.

Grazier notes that economic research supports offering physicians financial incentives to promote behavior change, but we are unable to discern such an effect from data reported with the case. However, the case reports that primary care physicians were, in the end, motivated by the professional confidence that they were making the correct clinical interventions, "without regard for remuneration."

The research question was inspired by published literature estimating that depression will be the second most common disease worldwide by 2020. In the context of EB management, the findings appear to be actionable, particularly in the context of large, self-insured employers or traditional health maintenance organizations, but follow-up is needed. As noted by Grazier, the business case is a work in progress. "While the improvements in the clinical depression scores among case subjects were noteworthy, the study could not directly translate these into cost savings for employers." At the *management* frontier, this is likely to be a rather unequivocal go/no-go decision point that divides spirited EB management from the more rarified realm of experimentation.

Results of EB management: By analyzing medical and systems management and health economics, physician managers were able to implement a process aimed at improving the care of depression patients. The literature had already demonstrated the need for champions at each clinic, well-trained staff and providers, a computerized patient registry system, shared medical and mental health information, communication across all lines, and documentation of clinical outcomes and direct/indirect costs.

Data-Driven Inpatient Bed Planning (page 189)

Problem: A large academic medical center was functioning at 86 percent inpatient bed utilization, resulting in scheduling difficulties, emergency department diversion, and other operational issues. Trends suggested that demand for inpatient beds would continue to grow.

Research question: How can a hospital evaluate and realign inpatient beds to better meet the organization's current and future needs?

Comment: Jancy Strauman's case examines bed capacity constraints in a large quaternary academic medical center with growing inpatient volume. Using internal data, a model for forecasting utilization trends with interactive assumptions, and a demand analysis, the study created a bed utilization plan capable of meeting current needs and supporting strategic growth. This transparent, data-driven process allowed key stakeholders, such as clinical department chiefs, to view the demand assumptions and understand the evidence-based rationale for unit redesignations; to create new resources such as step-down beds; and to grapple with guidelines for bed access and assignment. Finally, the process unmasked how some root causes of current bed shortages, including physician scheduling and long patient lengths of stay, exacerbated both the current emergency and future bed shortages.

The research question was framed appropriately for a hospital confronting an immediate emergency situation as well as planning for the future. Benchmarking its utilization patterns with those of other organizations also would have been useful, particularly with regard to length-of-stay trends and the relationship of certain types of beds, such as multi-bed rooms and the availability of step-down beds, to overall utilization. The hospital's own internal demand data were the primary and most important data source for actionable recommendations.

This hospital's length-of-stay pattern has a profound, distortive effect on creating actionable bed-need scenarios. Management needs to understand better what drives this pattern and, more important, the steps being taken to address it, before costly bed resources are dedicated to what may be inherent inefficiency. Management also must examine how the "right" number of beds is being determined and updated.

Results of EB management: This case demonstrates the important role internal evidence can play in management decisions. Evaluating past utilization trends and conducting a demand analysis enabled the hospital to plan how to meet its future needs. Evidence supported the creation of bed stack options that would foster other strategic growth initiatives. Besides addressing the immediate issue, evidence also suggested what to expect if the hospital could not execute the solution effectively.

Using Evidence-Based Management to Improve Operating Room Scheduling (page 207)

Problem: Capacity challenges and expected continued growth forced operating room (OR) managers and clinical leadership to find a way to schedule OR time more efficiently.

Research questions: What is the current level of block utilization, what is the variation among departments, and what opportunities exist for improving overall utilization and minimizing interdepartmental variation?

Comment: This case, by Megin Wolfman, addresses the problem of growing utilization in a capacity-challenged operating room environment in a major academic medical center. By framing the research questions appropriately, and at fairly low costs, the hospital was able to create OR utilization profiles by department and an interactive database that could fairly reallocate block time among departments on the basis of utilization. Because physicians are data and evidence driven, the EB management approach enabled major change to occur in an apolitical manner and avoided a turf battle based on anecdote, incomplete information, and opinion. Preliminary results were positive, in that departments whose block time was reallocated experienced significant gains in efficiency and utilization during the first review cycle.

It would have been interesting to benchmark this hospital against others to determine whether efficiency comparisons could be made. It would also be interesting to see whether efficiency improvements are sustained over time, since Wolfman believes the reallocation model "holds longer-term promise of improved efficiency and profitability and effective capacity creation." Can physicians "game" the system? Are there perverse incentives associated with a "use it or lose it" mind-set for block booking? Finally, how does the model address the variability among physicians who take dramatically different amounts of time for relatively similar cases? Can it help narrow these differences, or does it just perpetuate the status quo? All these questions are important as hospital management continues to adapt and refine this model.

Results of EB management: Management was able to cost-effectively identify varying OR utilization patterns across clinical departments, enabling development of immediate solutions to accommodate growing demand. In addition, evidence enabled creation of an efficient and fair method of reallocating OR block time.

Evidence-Based Criteria for Hospital Evacuation: The Case of Hurricane Katrina (page 219)

Problem: The issues faced by hospitals in the aftermath of Hurricane Katrina—role confusion, poor coordination, inadequate communication, lack of integrated planning—have motivated many facilities to reassess their emergency preparedness plans.

Research question: Do hospitals have an effective, systematic, and evidence-based plan for evacuation in the event of a disaster, and if so, what are the criteria for determining that and how are they used?

Comment: The case, by K. Joanne McGlown and colleagues, explores the response of New Orleans hospitals to Hurricane Katrina, examines past response performance, and poses questions about how hospitals can plan more effectively for the future. Research questions could have been framed somewhat differently, such as: How did New Orleans medical centers plan for the Katrina disaster? How can such planning and disaster response be accomplished more effectively in the future, given acceptable cost constraints? Determining what defines acceptable costs and who pays them are key parts of the disaster planning challenge, which also require organizations to define the outcome sought: zero casualties? Or zero *avoidable* casualties? What are the trade-offs among the alternative desired outcomes and their acceptability under various conditions?

In this case study, the authors focus on New Orleans hospitals' poor planning for patient evacuations before Katrina. Clearly, a lack of preparedness for potential evacuation placed patients at risk. As the authors point out, a basic problem in healthcare disaster planning is unfunded mandates. From the manager's point of view, costs of planning are borne by specific institutions, but benefits are distributed widely across other organizations and the general public and may not be realized for years, or decades. Thus, the hospital manager's responsibility must be limited, for example, to ensuring that current patients are properly cared for. The manager should inform public authorities about planning the hospital has done and what it cannot do adequately because of lack of funding and other reasons.

Results of EB management: EB management can reduce variability in the planning process, thereby improving the quality of the plan. Successful evidence-based planning for emergencies means all managers learn to pay attention to the same critical issues, halt poor practices, and increase adoption of best practices.

Improving the Health Status of Underserved Children in Houston's East End (page 233)

Problem: Charities wanted to find a way to help an underserved neighborhood with unmet public health needs.

Research question: What is the best way to assess the health status of children in an underserved neighborhood in Houston?

Comment: Patricia Bray describes the interventions of a charitable foundation in the East End neighborhood of Houston. The Episcopal Health Charities were incorporated "to integrate philanthropy with community-based research through an evidence-based management approach." The project is well-grounded in empirical evidence, partly due to the close interaction of the charity and the University of Texas School of Public Health, Houston. This interaction demonstrates the opportunity for more isolated practice environments to receive assistance with literature reviews, databases, and research methodology.

Of particular note in the East End project is a program design that incorporates "colloquial and research-based" evidence. Along with customary primary and secondary data sources, structured input from the underserved population was used to score possible interventions. The project posted data on the Web using data mapping software, which made baseline data and intervention results readily available to others. Thus, the researchers created an intentional Hawthorne effect, raising community awareness and generating participatory interest.

This case is a strong example of the potential impact of EB management in the health sector. Project leadership has grown from the research, rather than the management, side of a complex organization, which suggests that large health systems may benefit from internal development of certain skill sets.

Results of EB management: The EB management process enabled Episcopal Health Charities to break down its overall research question into smaller, more manageable queries. Assessing the evidence focused the researchers' efforts by clearly identifying pressing public health needs, resulting in improved community health status.

Reference

Berwick, D. 2007. "Eating Soup with a Fork." Keynote address, 19th National Forum on Quality Improvement in Health Care, December 11. Available at: www.ihi.org/IHI/Programs/AudioAnd WebPrograms /OnDemandPresentationBerwick.htm.

LEADERSHIP DEVELOPMENT AT THE SAINT BONIFACE HEALTHCARE SYSTEM

Philip DiSalvio

Introduction

Betty Arthur reflected on the crucial and complicated issue of leadership development at the Saint Boniface Healthcare System and wondered whether the system's leadership development initiative was all it could be. As the vice president of human resource development of the largest healthcare system in one of the Northeast's most populous states, Arthur is charged with creating a system-wide learning environment to ensure that a succession of qualified candidates is available to lead the organization in the years ahead, especially as the system faces increasing competitive challenges.

The Saint Boniface Healthcare System (SBHCS), the state's second-largest private employer, has more than 22,000 employees, 4,750 physicians (representing one-fourth of the total physicians actively practicing in the state), and 443 residents. Each year, it serves more than 2 million patients, including 225,000 inpatients and same-day surgery patients, 450,000 emergency department patients, and 1.5 million outpatients, and delivers more than 17,500 babies.

The state's largest integrated healthcare delivery system, SBHCS comprises seven acute care hospitals, nine nursing and rehabilitation centers, several outpatient facilities, a large ambulatory healthcare center, two assisted living facilities, a psychiatric hospital, a center for gynecological surgery, and a comprehensive hospice, home care, and behavioral health network. It is managed by a skilled Senior Corporate Management Group (Figure 10.1). Although located in a highly competitive geographic area, SBHCS commands sizable market share. But shifting market forces, government program cuts, the growing number of uninsured, a widening gap in charity funding, mounting competition posed by new niche facilities, and an array of other forces have put its market advantage increasingly at risk.

FIGURE 10.1
Saint Boniface
Healthcare
System Table of
Organization

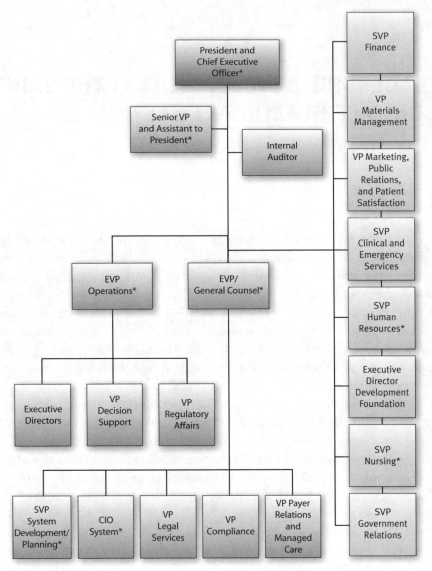

*Senior Corporate Management Group

Arthur considered SBHCS a contemporary model for the "sacred business" of healthcare and was thankful that its president/CEO was committed to SBHCS's human resource–driven philosophy and core values:

- Quality care
- Employee/patient/physician/resident satisfaction
- Responsible financial management
- Execution
- Sustainability

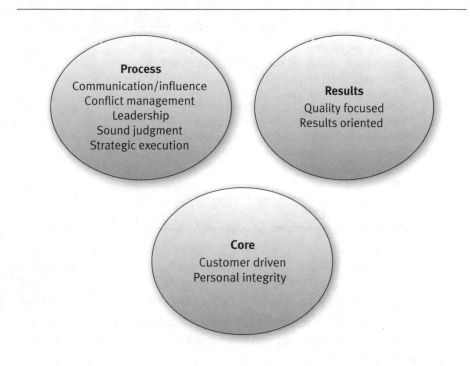

FIGURE 10.2
Saint Boniface
Healthcare
System
Department
Head/
Director–Level
Competency
Model

The SBHCS Leadership Institute

The SBHCS Leadership Institute embodied its ethos with its focus on leadership competencies. In 1997, management hired an independent consultant to facilitate development of a leadership competency model (Figure 10.2). The consultant worked with the system's executive directors—the chief administrators of SBHCS's various facilities, who report directly to the executive vice president of operations—and with corporate members of senior management, who have system-wide responsibility for certain key functions and report directly to the president/CEO.

The competency model emphasized core attributes, process skills, and achievement of results. Using it as their foundation, corporate senior management recruited a group of thought leaders from inside and outside SBHCS to create a leadership development curriculum, akin to a "mini executive MBA." They engaged healthcare management faculty members from several universities to work with the consultant and senior management to launch what ultimately became known as the SBHCS Leadership Institute.

The first SBHCS Leadership Institute, held in September 1998, involved 30 individuals from the system. Participants were nominated by their respective executive director or vice president. The human resource development office made the final selection, targeting managers with high potential and, in some cases, people who recently had been promoted.

Box 10.1
Saint Boniface
Healthcare
System
Leadership
Institute
Program
Modules

Half-Day Program Modules
1. SBHCS Core Values and Management Expectations
2. Leadership Skills and Versatility
3. Driving Change
4. Human Resources/People Strategy
5. Managing in Today's Healthcare Environment
6. Strategic Decision Making and Implementation
7. Financial Management for the Healthcare Manager
8. Effective Use of Information
9. Achieving Quality Excellence
10. Maintaining a Customer-Driven Environment
11. Cultural Diversity
12. Marketing and Maintaining Competitive Advantage

From 1998 to 2002, the Leadership Institute was held semiannually. After 2003 budget exigencies compelled a cutback. The Leadership Institute was pared down to an annual event. Structured around six all-day sessions, the program curriculum included a dozen half-day "courses" (Box 10.1).

Missed Goals

Feedback about the Leadership Institute from participants and senior corporate management was consistently positive. Nonetheless, Arthur began to have misgivings. She thought the Institute's curriculum and methods might have relied too heavily on "internal wisdom," that is, what senior corporate management and external experts considered required content for leadership development—priorities built on consensus, instinct, tradition, and individual experience. But Arthur's primary worry was whether the Institute was producing the intended outcomes. Available data reinforced her concern:

- Of the 488 individuals who had attended the Leadership Institute since 1998, 59 percent of those still on staff had not advanced in the organization.
- At the end of 2006, just under half of new managers were recruited through internal promotion (47 percent); the rest were new hires.
- A study by SBHCS's Human Resource Department indicated that only 16 percent of its current management pool was considered ready for advancement.

   Clearly, the Leadership Institute needed to reexamine whether it was achieving its original purposes, from two perspectives: (1) were the leadership competencies established in the original competency model still relevant; and (2) if they were, was the Leadership Institute's curriculum actually strengthening them? Arthur was committed to pursuing these goals, perceiving people as the only assets with the adaptive power to sustain organizational success, and effective leadership as one of the most powerful competitive advantages an organization can possess. Reexamining the Leadership Institute made strong business sense.

A Systematic Process for Evaluating Alternatives

Arthur needed a systematic process to examine these issues. She thought she might learn from a movement that had taken the medical establishment a long way toward grounding clinical decisions on the latest and best knowledge: evidence-based medicine. A similar approach might aid management decision making. Arthur recognized that this approach would have to incorporate the considerable experience, talent, and knowledge of individuals in SBHCS. To complement their contributions and to help ensure a more objective, data-driven strategy, she also wanted to bring in the best available evidence on leadership development.

Consideration of what exactly constituted "evidence" called to mind the kind of evidence that originally had been used to create the Leadership Institute—internal wisdom—which included tacit knowledge held by the senior corporate leadership team, the executive directors, and the external consultants. The competencies, structure, and content of the Leadership Institute had been based on this knowledge, which included opinions and personal perspectives on how leaders should respond in various situations. This type of evidence had some clear strengths. In particular, it took into account the context, resources, structure, culture, and decision-making capabilities of SBHCS—crucial elements in a viable leadership development strategy.

But Arthur saw that this internal wisdom needed to be balanced with a more systematic, empirical approach that would increase the Leadership Institute's credibility and perhaps make the program more relevant and results oriented. To redesign SBHCS's leadership initiatives, she would need research evidence, obtained through the systematic collection and analysis of trends, practice patterns, and outcomes.

Applying an Evidence-Based Management Approach

In taking a fresh look at leadership development at SBHCS, Arthur considered the best possible way to implement an evidence-based approach. The literature described a six-step process that applied evidence to the assessment and selection of the "best" alternatives.

Step 1: Formulating the Research Question

Plainly, a relevant and up-to-date leadership competency model and methods for enhancing those competencies were needed. Arthur knew that the management literature on the topic was overwhelming. A Google search

FIGURE 10.3
Sources of
Evidence

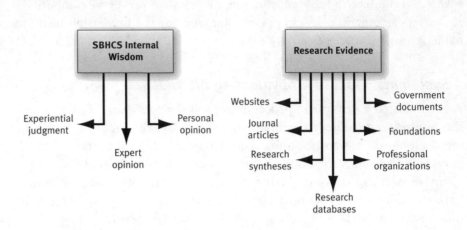

on "leadership development" produced more than 1.5 million entries. She would have to frame the issue and refine her queries in a way that would increase her chance of locating the specific, most relevant research.

The search query "Which leadership development option is better?" was too broad, vague, and abstract. Narrower questions, focused on outcomes, particularly evidence comparing outcomes within a similar context, would serve better. With these criteria in mind, Arthur devised the following research questions: What competencies among SBHCS's senior decision makers would likely increase their succession readiness? What mechanisms for enhancing those competencies produce the best leadership succession readiness outcomes?

With these questions clearly in mind, Arthur was ready to look for evidence that might provide some answers.

Step 2: Acquiring Research Information

SBHCS had recently made significant investments in its knowledge management resources, and Arthur considered the array of resources she might tap. She knew she had to seek the best research available and integrate that information with the extensive internal wisdom on hand at SBHCS.

The SBHCS Medical Library was accessible 24 hours a day and staffed by four medical librarians. It contained 5,500 textbooks and monographs, 15,500 bound journals, and 425 current journal subscriptions. Computer-assisted literature searches of National Library of Medicine databases were available. The library also was a member of a statewide information network. New computer workstations featured the Medical Literature Analysis and Retrieval System and interactive knowledge management programs. Internet access on Arthur's office computer, and the in-office corporate webmaster and director of decision support, also could help her track down the right information.

Arthur soon realized that there might be just too much evidence. To organize her thoughts, she visualized the sources of information at her disposal and constructed a diagram of those she might reasonably consult for help (Figure 10.3). Then, with her understanding of the resources available and the sources of evidence she might use, Arthur had to develop a search strategy. Wanting to avoid research "blind alleys," she contacted the Medical Library. The librarian explained that the choice of research tool would depend on the kind of information Arthur was seeking:

- If Arthur was simply trying to learn what was available in the subject area, she could start by selecting a Yahoo! subject directory. Subject directories, unlike search engines, are created and maintained by human editors, rather than electronic spiders or robots. Subject editors review and select sites for inclusion in their directories on the basis of various selection criteria, and the resources they list are usually annotated.
- Alternatively, if Arthur wanted to look for a specific piece of information, she could use a major search engine, such as Google, or a specialized database. The librarian explained that search engines are large databases that have been assembled electronically. Individual search engines compile their own searchable databases.
- If Arthur wanted to retrieve everything on the subject, she could try the same search on several search engines. These "metasearches" hunt the databases of multiple search engines simultaneously.
- Finally, she could use resources available in the library in hard copy, such as books, newspapers, journals, and other print references.

Using the Internet to Acquire Research Evidence
Considering the vast and readily accessible information at her disposal, and given time and resource constraints, Arthur settled on two Internet searches to acquire the research evidence she needed on leadership competencies and mechanisms that produce the best results for succession readiness:

- A web search for systematic reviews and meta-analyses that synthesized relevant research articles and
- A bibliographic database search for relevant published and unpublished primary studies.

The search for systematic reviews and meta-analyses of relevant research found only two articles related to managerial leadership development. The more helpful was a 2002 meta-analysis entitled "The Effectiveness of Managerial Leadership Development Programs: A Meta-Analysis of Studies from 1982–2001," the doctoral dissertation of Doris B. Collins. In it, Collins synthesized 103 existing studies involving a broad range of settings, researchers, and circumstances and a full range of managerial leadership development interventions. She integrated conflicting findings and established a general knowledgebase about managerial leadership development. Collins concluded that the relationship between leadership development and performance was not clear.

Then, using meta-analytic techniques, Collins integrated results of 83 studies involving formal training interventions to determine their effectiveness (enhancement of performance, knowledge, and expertise at the individual, team or group, and organizational levels). Collins's meta-analysis showed that the effectiveness of managerial leadership development programs varied widely. However, she concluded that if organizations offered the right development programs to the right people at the right time, they could feel comfortable that their leadership development programs could produce positive results. In other words, her research showed that the content of the most effective training programs was driven by the organization's strategic framework.

The bibliographic database search provided several leads. Arthur's search included:

- The National Library of Medicine Gateway—622 citations
- Google Scholar—304 citations for "leadership development outcomes"
- MEDLINE and PubMed—3,627 citations for "leadership development" and 32 for "leadership competencies"
- ProQuest—1 citation for "leadership competencies and healthcare"

Keyword searches including both "leadership" and "succession readiness" revealed no primary research studies but returned many "expert opinions."

Among the most promising research articles found using keywords of "healthcare leadership competencies" and "healthcare leadership development" were the following:

- A Delphi analysis of six studies that identified essential areas of management expertise, including leadership competencies, required for future healthcare executives (Hudak, Brooke Jr., and Finstuen 2000)
- Another Delphi analysis predicting the job skills, knowledge, and abilities necessary for successful healthcare management in the future (Sentell and Finstuen 1998)
- A study in which 30 health system CEOs and 15 early careerists evaluated a list of technical, interpersonal, and strategic competencies as to their relevance in real-life situations, which revealed useful depth and detail about managers' educational needs (Griffith et al. 2002)
- A study involving key informant interviews and a literature review that identified competencies critical to early careerists' preparation for advancement (Specific work experiences and academic courses were mapped to each competency, indicating where and how the competency might be developed [Robbins, Bradley, and Spicer 2001].)

- An eight-year evaluation of an effective year-long leadership development program serving senior public health leaders, which created a leadership development model relevant to healthcare administrators in general (Woltring, Constantine, and Schwarte 2003)

Professional Organizations

Database searches of professional healthcare-related websites also revealed
promising leads. Arthur found that the National Center for Healthcare
Leadership (NCHL) had conducted extensive research on healthcare leadership competencies. This research included examination of new expectations for individual behavior and organizational performance critical to
meeting the Institute of Medicine's goals for improving the nation's healthcare system. These leadership competencies had been benchmarked against
the nation's leading healthcare organizations, as well as top-performing
organizations outside the health sector. According to NCHL President
Marie E. Sinioris:

> We know from research and experiences of other industries that excel-
> lent leadership is a key differentiator in the performance of organiza-
> tions...by researching the behaviors and best practices of leadership
> development from the top-performing organizations in the Fortune
> 100, and adapting these behaviors and best practices to the health
> industry, we are breaking new ground and raising the bar for health
> management professionals and for educators in the field. These com-
> petencies are critical to NCHL's mission to improve organizational
> performance by improving leadership.

The NCHL website also addressed the validity of its competency model:

> With the validation of the competency model by the Hay Group, Inc.,
> a global human resources company that has studied competency mod-
> eling for more than 40 years, NCHL will begin implementing the Health
> Leadership Competency Model in demonstration projects in both uni-
> versity and health system settings.

Arthur found another promising lead related to succession planning
in a 2004 report, "CEO Succession Planning in Freestanding U.S.
Hospitals," on the website of the American College of Healthcare Executives
(ACHE). Researchers conducted a national survey to determine the current state of practice in hospital CEO succession planning. The survey was
constructed from a review of succession planning research and practice
writings to determine the extent to which current practices reflected "best
practices." CEOs and board chairs were queried, and 722 institutions
responded (a 44 percent response rate).

The survey results revealed widespread agreement that succession planning is a valuable and important strategy for hospitals, but they also exposed substantial variation in practice. In terms of candidate development, the most powerful activities appeared to be mentoring and assignments. The data also suggested that the greater the number of developmental activities employed, the higher the perceived effectiveness of the process.

External Healthcare Systems as a Source of Evidence

Arthur also attempted to learn more about leadership development initiatives of other healthcare systems. She obtained a list of similar-sized health systems from the American Hospital Association and sent their human resource development departments a questionnaire about their leadership competency model and the type and format of their leadership development programs. She also requested data on their promotion results. Knowing that some of this information might be considered proprietary, Arthur did not expect many replies, and, in fact, she received none.

Internal Wisdom as a Source of Evidence

Arthur recalled her "sources of evidence" diagram and proposed that research gathered internally also might provide information relevant to her research questions. She constructed a survey tool for use in conjunction with a series of focus groups involving board members, senior corporate executives, executive directors, and other key senior staff. Using the Delphi method, she collected data from these groups regarding elements of leadership competency models and delivery methods they believed would produce both high succession readiness levels and the best leadership succession outcomes. Arthur also hoped that this internal research would facilitate formation of a collective judgment, which would be helpful later in implementing strategies informed by her research.

Step 3: Assessing the Validity, Quality, and Applicability of the Evidence

While Arthur believed that her hunt for research evidence had uncovered some useful information, she knew that all evidence is not equal. If she were to justify a revised and more up-to-date competency model and recommend a new approach to leadership development, she knew she would have to demonstrate its direct relation to increased levels of succession readiness with useful, high-quality evidence.

Certain characteristics related to usefulness came to mind, and Arthur knew that these characteristics would have to be applied to both internal wisdom and primary research. She compiled a set of anticipated questions

FIGURE 10.4
Quality and
Usefulness
Assessment of
Evidence

Quality of Evidence	Ranking		
Strength of the research design			
Applicability to context and setting of SBHCS			
Characteristics of the study groups			
Measurement reliability and validity			
Methodology used			
Supportability of the data to the conclusions			
Author of the study			
Consistency of the data with other studies			
Cumulative score ranking			
Usefulness of Evidence	Ranking		
Accuracy of the evidence			
Relevance of the evidence			
Application of the evidence to implementation			
Accessibility of the evidence			
Cumulative score ranking			

Rankings of quality
1 = Poor
2 = Fair
3 = Good

Rankings of usefulness
1 = Not very useful
2 = Moderately
    useful
3 = Very useful

about these two types of evidence: (1) Is the evidence accurate? (2) Is it relevant? (3) Can it be applied within the context of SBHCS? (4) Is it readily obtainable? (For example, Arthur may have learned that other healthcare systems have well-regarded leadership development initiatives, but could she find out more about them?)

Once she established these usefulness criteria, Arthur thought about how to gauge the quality of the evidence she had amassed. Recalling her graduate course in research methods, she listed basic parameters that would help her assess the quality of the management research. Arthur then assembled her usefulness and quality indicators into a rankings matrix (Figure 10.4).

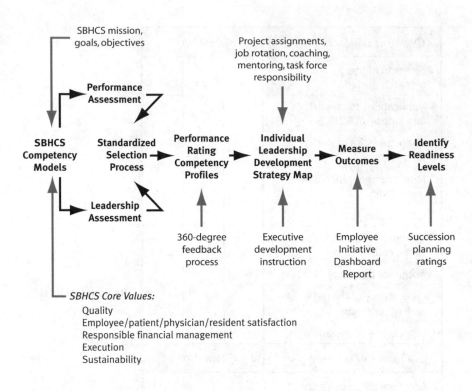

Step 4: Presenting the Evidence

Finally, Arthur prepared to present the evidence. To avoid any perception of selective citation or information bias, she organized an evidence assessment task force consisting of representative members of the board, senior corporate management, and the executive directors. This group appreciated the breadth and depth of Arthur's research and used the criteria established in the rankings matrix to assess its usefulness and quality. Specifically, the task force examined the results of the Internet searches (the meta-analyses), the bibliographic databases (pertinent research articles, NCHL, and ACHE), and the internal Delphi survey/focus groups. After compiling their scores and drawing together the highest-ranked evidence, the task force recommended what they considered the most relevant leadership competency models and then summarized this evidence for the senior corporate management group.[1]

Feedback from Senior Corporate Management

Although the evidence assessment task force analysis and research data rankings had increased awareness of various studies and findings, Arthur considered the potential difficulty in persuading senior corporate management to apply that evidence to an updated leadership development intervention. Several senior managers stipulated that outcomes had to be the driving force behind any intervention's design and implementation. Others were concerned about the need to connect competencies to the system's core values. Still others believed that succession planning and future leadership could not rely exclusively on a series of "leadership seminars."

As a result, the senior corporate management group directed the task force to consider a leadership development and succession initiative that would do more than merely modify the leadership competency model or change the format and content of the Leadership Institute. Instead, they asked for a systematic plan incorporating:

- The alignment of a leadership competency model with the organization's strategic vision;
- An assessment system that would measure leadership potential;
- Measurement of outcomes of leadership development interventions; and
- A multifaceted leadership succession readiness approach.

Step 5: Applying the Evidence to the Decision

Much of what the senior corporate management group advised had been suggested in the research evidence regarding effective outcomes—that is, a systems approach to succession planning and leadership development and a tight link to organizational strategy. Arthur asked the task force to stay in operation and help shape this ambitious new initiative. Incorporating the senior managers' recommendations, the task force revisited and analyzed the research evidence and crafted a systems approach to leadership development and succession planning. The result was the SBHCS Leadership Development and Succession Planning Process (Figure 10.5).

Using the research evidence on leadership competency models—especially that cited by NCHL—the task force devised a model for leadership development and succession planning that incorporated SBHCS's core values, mission, goals, and objectives. They developed a selection process and criteria for managers who would be invited to participate in a leadership track. These individuals would undergo a 360-degree feedback process and receive a leadership competency profile including performance metrics and a specific, individually tailored leadership development strategy map. The map would include project assignments, coaching, and assignment of a mentor. It also would list the trainee's responsibilities in working with the task force and committees and in executive development instruction (Figure 10.6).

Outcomes, in terms of job movement, organizational advancement, and indicators of readiness, would be measured and compiled in the Employee Initiative Dashboard Report. This report would figure heavily

FIGURE 10.6
SBHCS
Leadership
Development
Strategy Map
Model

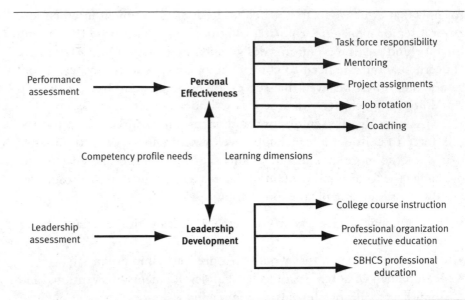

Performance assessment → **Personal Effectiveness**

- Task force responsibility
- Mentoring
- Project assignments
- Job rotation
- Coaching

Competency profile needs   Learning dimensions

Leadership assessment → **Leadership Development**

- College course instruction
- Professional organization executive education
- SBHCS professional education

in identifying a pool of individuals as potential successors to key leadership positions in SBHCS and provide data for assessing the leadership development initiative itself.

Step 6: Evaluating Results

With the approval of the senior corporate management group, Arthur planned to launch the SBHCS Leadership Development and Succession Planning Process as a two-year pilot project in one of the system's hospitals. A pilot project made sense, not only because of the investment in time and resources that would be dedicated to such a project, but for the necessary close monitoring and inevitable fine-tuning.

As she prepared to roll out her presentation on the pilot to the selected hospital's key staff, Arthur reflected on the risk in introducing widespread organizational change at SBHCS, as in all large, complex organizations. However, the evidence-based approach she had used to support the leadership development intervention reassured her that SBHCS had made the best, most informed decision possible.

Endnote

1. This group comprises the president/chief executive officer, the senior vice president and assistant to the president, the executive vice president of operations, the executive vice president/general counsel, the chief information officer of the system, the senior vice president of system

development and planning, the senior vice president of nursing, and the senior vice president of human resources.

References

Griffith, J. R., G. L. Warden, K. Neighbors, and B. Shim. 2002. "A New Approach to Assessing Skill Needs of Senior Managers." *The Journal of Health Administration Education* 20 (1): 75–98.

Hudak, R. P., P. P. Brooke Jr., and K. Finstuen. 2000. "Identifying Management Competencies For Healthcare Executives: Review Of A Series Of Delphi Studies." *The Journal of Health Administration Education* 18(2) 13-43.

Robbins, C. J., E. H. Bradley, and M. Spicer. 2001. "Developing Leadership in Healthcare Administration: A Competency Assessment Tool/Practitioner Application." *Journal of Healthcare Management* 46(3): 188–202.

Sentell, J. W., and K. Finstuen. 1998. "Executive Skills 21: A Forecast of Leadership Skills and Associated Competencies Required by Naval Hospital Administrators into the 21st Century." *Military Medicine* 163 (1): 3–8.

Woltring, C., W. Constantine, and L. Schwarte. 2003. "Does Leadership Training Make a Difference? The CDC/UC Public Health Leadership Institute: 1991–1999." *Journal of Public Health Management & Practice* 9 (2): 103–22.

FORMING A CORPORATE UNIVERSITY: MORE OF THE SAME, OR SOMETHING NEW?

Ann Scheck McAlearney

Introduction

"How come every time we need a new department manager, we have to recruit someone from outside our organization? Don't we spend plenty of money on training and development here?" complained Grace Long to her executive team. Long, chief executive officer of Best Health System, was frustrated with the numbers she was seeing.

Best Health System is considered one of the premier health systems in its Midwest market area. Comprising six hospitals, a home health company, and a large group of ambulatory care centers, Best Health enjoys an excellent reputation, often overshadowing the local academic medical center.

Recently, however, several health system executives expressed concern about the preparedness of newly promoted managers and supervisors. Further, they believed that too many departments were trying to do the same things, and they sensed that this duplication added costs without taking advantage of system-wide strengths. For instance, leadership training for nurse managers was offered in four different settings: (1) at each hospital through individual nursing departments; (2) on-site through a local university; (3) by the organizational development department; and (4) by the Process Excellence Department.

Lily Green, system vice president for organizational development, heard the urgency in these complaints. Green had been working at Best Health for the past year and knew that the results of Best Health's training and development programs should look much better. Having come from another industry, she had spent much of the past 12 months masking her surprise about how "behind" healthcare seemed to be in human resources and organizational development. Now, though, hearing Long's frustration and aware of other executives' concerns, Green sensed opportunity.

On the way back to her office, Green started considering possibilities for making major changes in employee training and development at Best Health. While there were several options, her mind kept coming back to one intriguing approach: What if a corporate university could be developed at

Best Health? There had been corporate universities in her last two companies, and she saw no reason why she couldn't explore this option at Best Health. She decided that the best way to answer this question and to craft a general strategy to improve staff development would be to use the six-step process of evidence-based management. This process would provide the sound evidence the executive team and Best Health board would need to make decisions about employee training and development that would likely affect most of the Best Health workforce.

Applying Evidence-Based Management

Step 1: Formulating the Research Question

While largely unknown within the healthcare industry, the trend toward organizing education and development programs using a corporate university model was making headlines across the country. General Electric's (GE) famed Crotonville Learning Center in Ossining, NY, (see www.ge.com/en/company/companyinfo/welchcenter/welch.htm), had been recently renamed the John F. Welch Leadership Center in honor of the company's legendary former CEO, who ascribed much of GE's success to careful attention to leadership development. And Green had always liked the concept behind McDonald's Corporation's "Hamburger U." in Oakbrook Terrace, IL (see www.mcdonalds.com/usa/work/m_careers/training.html), where the company trained a diverse group of managers in the McDonald's way. Disney was also ahead of the game, as she learned when visiting the Disney Institute as part of a conference in Orlando, Florida.

But Best Health was nothing like Disney or McDonald's. Best Health provided healthcare services, working with community physicians who weren't even employees and satisfying the many competing priorities of its diverse stakeholders—patients, insurers, board members, and employees. Yet, were there parallels?

As Green started to think about how the model might work, she became excited—and anxious. After a full year at Best Health, she knew a proposal to develop something as "fringe" as a corporate university would receive plenty of flak. For starters, just the word *corporate* in the project title would make many of the long-term employees hyperventilate. Also, some of the system's leaders might reject the concept of their employer as some sort of "university." Despite her misgivings, Green knew a corporate university had tremendous potential. She just had to collect the evidence and make her case.

Step 2: Searching for Evidence

Green's first step was an Internet search for information about leading corporate universities. Green and her administrative fellow, Molly Miller, rapidly filled a binder with web printouts. Since information available on the web varies in quality, Miller began a formal literature review. Using search terms such as "corporate university," "leadership development," "executive education," and "management training," Miller found published articles and books that provided valuable information.

In little time, they had accumulated more pages of information than they could easily manage. Miller offered to create a searchable database to organize the information and help guide their investigation. As the database grew, so did their list of questions. How hard was it to develop a corporate university? How much did it cost? How long did it take? Was it even possible in a healthcare organization? Putting their list of questions together, the two decided that their next step would be to interview some of the organizations that intrigued them the most.

Miller's experience in her MHA program had exposed her to several research methods, and one that seemed particularly appropriate for this purpose was the structured interview. She and Green created a list of target organizations to form a purposeful sample and then crafted a list of questions to guide the interviews. By asking the same questions across multiple interviews, Green and Miller would add validity to the evidence they were gathering. They organized the list of questions (Box 11.1) into five major topics:

- A description of the corporate university being studied
- The program implementation process
- Barriers and facilitators to program development and implementation
- Program evaluation
- Program evolution

Armed with these questions, Green and Miller had to decide how they wanted to focus their interviews. Were they curious only about how the healthcare field was upgrading its staff educational efforts, or did they want to continue to look outside their industry? Given the quantity of literature they had reviewed, the two believed they had a good idea about what was going on in other industries, but they had found almost no information about what hospitals and health systems were doing. They decided to narrow their investigation to healthcare organizations and to learn as much as possible about those considered leaders in the field.

Framing this study as a search for best practices enabled Green to develop a formal proposal she could take to the CEO. Armed with the results of their background literature search, Green and Miller wrote a brief proposal seeking funds and time to study corporate universities in U.S. healthcare organizations and to visit five that they would identify as having model programs. They decided to make this site identification process part of their research, building time into the initial phase of the project to assess and evaluate candidate organizations. Long rapidly approved their

Box 11.1

Sample
Interview Guide
for Studying
Corporate
Universities

Interview Questions

1. *Description of Corporate University*
   - Could you please describe the corporate university at this institution? (Get historical perspective.)
   - Why was the program initiated? When?
   - To whom/what is the program connected within the organization? Is the human resources department involved? (If so, how? How much?)
   - Does your corporate university outsource any services? What types?

2. *Program Implementation Process*
   - How was this program implemented in your organization?
   - What resources are needed for the program? What resources are allocated?
   - How are individuals selected to participate in the corporate university programs?

3. *Program Implementation: Barriers/Challenges and Facilitators*
   - What barriers have you/this program experienced in its introduction/implementation/continuance?
   - What strategies have you used to develop and promote the corporate university?

4. *Organizational Commitment and Program Evaluation*
   - How is leadership evaluated in this organization?
   - How is success/progress of the corporate university evaluated in this organization?
   - Who is accountable for the success or outcomes of the corporate university?

5. *Anticipated Program Enhancements/Changes*
   - How has the corporate university changed over time?
   - What changes/modifications are anticipated for the future?

plan but emphasized that their research should produce actionable information—that is, what Best Health would need to know to decide whether to invest in a corporate university.

Deepening Their Search

As a first step, Green and Miller produced a list of healthcare organizations they considered candidates for telephone interviews. There were ten. Miller then scheduled structured calls with key informants at each of the organizations and used an interview guide to frame her conversations. After every few calls, Miller met with Green to discuss her findings and raise new topics and questions. One question she asked each informant was, "Which healthcare organizations do you believe have model corporate universities that I should study?" Including this question allowed Miller to expand her initial sample, a technique called "snowball" sampling. In addition, as informants mentioned the same places time and again, she honed her list of site visit candidates.

After speaking with key informants at 20 organizations, Miller was confident that she had a good sense of what was going on with respect to corporate universities in healthcare and had a list of five organizations she thought would provide particularly informative site visits. With Green's approval, she contacted each of them, and she and Green cleared their calendars to hit the road.

The site visits exposed the small team to five very different organizations, but they were able to see in person both the places and the models they and their interviewees deemed best. By speaking to a broad group of key informants at each organization, they learned about the nuances of program design, development, implementation, and evaluation—all areas they would need to address if they wanted to introduce a corporate university at Best Health.

Returning home, Green and Miller put all they had learned from their visits and telephone interviews into the context of Best Health. Recalling the extensive strategic planning process Best Health had recently completed, Green consulted her copy of the organization's strategic plan. Using the strategic plan and its goals as a guide, Green and Miller reviewed their findings about corporate universities and composed a list of the knowledge and skills Best Health employees would need for the organization to execute this strategic plan successfully.

Armed with this list, their next step was clear: conduct a formal organizational assessment to determine what was going on at Best Health with respect to education, training, and development, and to identify any gaps in these areas.

Organizational Assessment at Best Health

Green and Miller again brainstormed topics and questions the organizational assessment should include. Their first set of questions was fairly straightforward and concerned the types of education and training then available through the Best Health system. However, they realized the answers to those questions could spark some fairly contentious political battles. When programs overlapped, which program would "win," and which would be replaced? Who would decide? When there were gaps, who would be in charge of filling them? Once they had a sense of the "lay of the land" at Best Health, they matched current offerings with current needs, as reflected in the strategic plan.

On the basis of all their research, a corporate university still seemed the best way to address current staff development priorities—and to position Best Health to respond to future needs. Now they had to create a specific plan for investment in this approach. This proposition raised new questions. Would a virtual corporate university or a bricks-and-mortar model be more appropriate at Best Health? What new programs would be proposed? How much would developing and implementing the selected corporate university model cost? What kinds of returns could they project? What would be the time frame? How would they incorporate a process to plan for the future? Heads spinning, they decided it was time to speak to Long again.

Step 3: Evaluating the Evidence Case

Green and Miller met with Long to review their findings and raise their questions. As Long listened quietly, she began to jot down questions of her own. The team seemed to have done a thorough search for information about corporate universities in healthcare, yet Long was not convinced that they had covered all the angles. Was the corporate university model possibly too narrow? What about other leadership and organizational development efforts that might not be called corporate universities? Further, given the relatively small number of organizations they had been able to study in healthcare, was their evidence valid? More important, could projections about program development at Best Health be extrapolated from this evidence?

Long decided the team needed to broaden its search and focus its analysis. First, she recommended that Green and Miller study several organizations outside of healthcare. While she did not know much about running a McDonald's franchise or manufacturing Toyotas, Long suspected that the team could learn a lot from talking to the experts who did.

Second, while she liked the corporate university model, she proposed that the team study several healthcare organizations that had well-recognized leadership development programs of different types. Even if the findings were slightly less focused, Long believed she would be more comfortable making an investment decision when she better understood the range of leadership development program opportunities.

Finally, Long proposed that Green and Miller also collect and organize information about the projected costs and benefits of implementing a corporate university model at Best Health. She acknowledged that some of this information might be difficult to obtain, but she challenged the team to develop a comprehensive business plan that she could use to justify the required investment to the health system's board and other stakeholders.

Green and Miller returned to Green's office excited about their charge. They recognized that, while they were convinced that a corporate university model was perfect for Best Health, the project could not succeed unless they could convince others of its value. With the next health system board meeting only a month away, they had to work fast.

Looking at their list of tasks, Green decided the work would be completed most efficiently by working on the different tasks at the same time, making sure they communicated well throughout the process. She placed Miller in charge of the broader search for evidence while she began an in-depth analysis of the evidence they had already collected.

Searching for More Evidence

Miller went back through her database and listed corporate universities in other industries. While she knew she might not be able to speak directly with the program directors or chief learning officers of each program, she was not shy, and she knew how to be creative in her search for evidence. Using various contacts and introductions, Miller developed a target list of 20 corporate universities outside the healthcare industry. Next, she developed a set of questions that would address gaps in the evidence she and Green had perceived from their initial interviews of healthcare organizations. Her first choice would be to hold in-depth interviews, similar to the ones she had had with healthcare industry informants, but, as an alternative, she also developed a brief written questionnaire she could e-mail or fax to potential informants (Box 11.2). In particular, she wanted information about corporate university costs, benefits, and utilization, as these topics would likely be of considerable interest to Best Health's key decision makers.

Meanwhile, Green began to work on the business plan. Knowing it would be most compelling if it painted a picture of opportunity based upon a solid strategic rationale, she was particularly concerned about the types of evidence they could and should include. Working with the data they had amassed, Green built a list of questions the plan had to address (Box 11.3). These questions were formulated around the five A's for assessing evidence for management decision making:

- **Availability**: Have I looked in the right places for the evidence?
- **Accuracy**: Is it valid, reliable, comprehensive, and from multiple perspectives?
- **Applicability**: Is it appropriate for the decision and for this organization?
- **Actionability**: What recommendations can be implemented on the basis of the evidence, and what intended and unintended consequences can be anticipated?
- **Adequacy**: Do I have enough information for Best Health to make its decision?

Examining each of these issues in detail, Green concluded that she and Miller had been satisfactorily thorough in their search for **available** evidence. While they had not been able to speak with everyone who had ever developed a corporate university in healthcare, they had reached "saturation," in that they had already spoken to everyone their interviewees suggested. Further, their search had been comprehensive, using multiple sources of information and multiple methods to seek that information (i.e., interviews, a questionnaire, literature searches, Internet searches, and so forth). They also had extended their search to consider organizations outside the healthcare industry and had considered additional programs in leadership development, as suggested by Long.

Box 11.2
Sample
Corporate
University
Questionnaire

Q. In the current fiscal year, approximately how much money is budgeted for your leadership development program?

    Enter sum: $ _____

Q. Compared to the previous fiscal year, is the budget this fiscal year (circle one):

    Less than last year 1

    About the same as last year. 2

    More than last year. 3

Q. How many full-time equivalents (FTEs) are associated with your leadership development program? (Include administrators, clerical help, etc.; do not include internal faculty.)

    Enter number of FTEs _____

Q. Does your system evaluate its leadership development program on the basis of its return on investment (ROI)?

    Yes . . . . 1 → Go to **Qa.**

    No. . . . . 2 → Skip to next **Q.**

    Don't know 3

    *Qa. If yes, what is the target ROI for the program?

        Enter percentage_____

    *Qb. What is the ROI for the program for the most recently available year?

        Enter percentage_____

Q. What is the scope of your program offerings (i.e., contact hours, classes, modules)?

    Enter number of hours _____

    Enter number of classes _____

    Enter number of modules _____

Q. Please indicate the origin of faculty for your leadership training program. How many instructors are employees of the organization, and how many are external to it?

    Internal instructors _____ Number _____ Proportion

    External instructors _____ Number _____ Proportion

          Total _____ Number 100%

Q. Following are some ways to **evaluate the effectiveness** of corporate university programs. Please indicate if any of these measures are used to demonstrate your program's effectiveness.

	In Effect	Being Developed	Not Used
Promotion rates	1	2	3
Employee job satisfaction	1	2	3
Succession planning	1	2	3
Turnover in unit led	1	2	3
Market share increase	1	2	3
Cost savings	1	2	3
Quality improvement	1	2	3

Other: Please list: _____

_____

Box 11.3
Assessing the
Five A's of
Evidence for
Corporate
Universities in
Healthcare
Organizations

Availability: Finding the Sources of Information (Have I looked in the right places for the evidence?)
- Investigating corporate universities in healthcare organizations
- Examining role of corporate universities in other industries
- Defining appropriate scope of a corporate university at this organization
  - What is going on now?
  - What gaps exist? (organizational needs assessment)
  - Virtual versus bricks-and-mortar models
- Determining costs and projected benefits of the corporate university
  - What will be replaced?
  - What will be new?
  - What is the time frame?
  - What is the vision for future development?

Accuracy: Assessing the Accuracy of the Information (Is it valid, reliable, comprehensive, from multiple perspectives?)
- Cost data
  - Development
  - Learning management system technology and tools
  - Staff
- Utilization projections
  - In-person courses
  - Online courses
  - Development programs
- Benefits projected
  - Defining benefits, perspectives of benefits (e.g., compliance education and documentation; employee opinion survey results)
  - Financial savings
  - Centralization of education and training
  - Reducing redundancy

Applicability: Assessing the Applicability of Information (for the decision and this organization)
- Issues surrounding data availability
- Issues about lack of best practices in healthcare organizations
- Issues about competing perspectives (e.g., human resources versus corporate; physicians versus administration)
- Issues about philosophical differences (e.g., cultural value of a learning organization versus saving money on training)

Actionability: Assessing the Actionability of Information (What recommendations can you implement with intended and unintended consequences?)
- What projections can be made with the available data?
- What short-term plans are recommended?
- What long-term plans are recommended?
- How do program recommendations fit with organizational strategy?
  - Whose opinions matter most?
  - How can the political process be influenced with evidence?

Adequacy: Determining Whether the Information Is Adequate (When do you have enough information to make your decision?)
- What gaps in the data exist?
- Is there sufficient information to build a business case in certain areas?
- Is a pilot program possible?
- What information must be reviewed after what period of time?
- Are organizational champions available to help with implementation?

SOURCE: Adapted with permission from *Journal of Healthcare Management* 52 (5): 335–341. Chicago: Health Administration Press, 2007.

When it came to **accuracy** of the evidence, Green had to admit she was not entirely sure. She believed the evidence they had gathered was valid, reliable, comprehensive, and from multiple perspectives, but she could not be completely confident that the projections she and Miller made about how a corporate university would evolve at Best Health would be accurate. As a consequence, she included sensitivity analyses in the business plan to assess the reasonableness of her assumptions.

With respect to **applicability**, Green knew their evidence was of mixed value. For instance, interviews they had held with small health systems comparable to Best Health seemed most applicable to their organization. However, some of the data they had obtained from larger systems, from for-profit entities, and from organizations in other industries were harder to apply. As an example, if a non-healthcare organization reported spending 2 percent of gross revenues per year on employee development, how did that figure translate to the Best Health environment? More important, if employee development activities included more than corporate university functions, how could those expense numbers be tied to corporate university results? Further, was 2 percent an appropriate target?

Green was again struck by how far behind healthcare organizations were compared to other industries with respect to organizational development programs and metrics to track program impact. Similar health systems had a limited number of best practices they could borrow. Green resolved that a corporate university developed at Best Health should take advantage of all the applicable evidence, regardless of industry, to move Best Health ahead of competing hospitals in employee and organizational development.

Yet another issue that became apparent in her consideration of the information's applicability was the perspective of their analysis. She knew there might be a stark contrast between the perspectives of corporate executives and the human resources department when asked about an appropriate target investment for the program, or even the reasonableness of calculating return on investment for a corporate university at all. Similarly, there were philosophical differences in the way individuals valued aspects of corporate universities. For instance, while a substantial group of employees might value learning and the cultural benefit of working within a learning organization, many in finance or the executive suite might see a corporate university primarily as a way to save money on training by reducing redundancy. Green was glad their data applied across perspectives and could support a balanced conversation about the prospects of the initiative.

Considering **actionability**, Green knew the evidence was actionable. She knew it would help management make a decision, and, if the decision were positive, it would contribute to the development and implementation of a solid plan for the corporate university. Their research enabled them to make projections about the development trajectory of a corporate university and to formulate specific plans for both the short and long term. In addition, Green knew Long would want to link their programmatic recommendations to organizational strategy at Best Health. She was fully aware that this linkage would be critical in obtaining Long's support for needed resources and solid positioning of the corporate university within the organization. Nonetheless, Green also knew the corporate culture of Best Health relied heavily on financial projections, and she sensed that their financials were perhaps the weakest component of their business case. Despite their search for evidence, they had been unable to calculate a solid return on investment projection from a corporate university in healthcare because none of the existing programs had yet demonstrated its value with this metric.

Finally, regarding the question of **adequacy**, Green was confident that they now had enough information for the board to make a decision.

Step 4: Presenting the Evidence

Analyses complete, Green and Miller set up six discrete decision options:

Option 1:   Doing nothing and maintaining the status quo

Option 2:   Developing a corporate university brand to label and include all current training and development activities now performed across the health system, without changing the structure or function of these activities

Option 3:   Outsourcing the corporate university function to a vendor of corporate university services and consulting

Option 4:   Contracting with a learning management system vendor for online courses only

Option 5:   Creating a new virtual Best Health corporate university that would include new technologies and organization-wide participation in resource allocation decisions regarding training and development activities

Option 6:   Building a new bricks-and-mortar Best Health corporate university at system headquarters to house learning and development opportunities at Best Health

Green and Miller made notes that would provide guidance in deciding among these alternatives. While they knew option 1 had to be presented, they were confident that Best Health's management did want to make a change of some kind. At the same time, they did not believe that Best Health had the surplus resources or political will to invest in option 6. Their research had led them to believe that option 2 was merely lip service to the concept of organizational learning and would be unlikely to achieve measurable improvement. In contrast, options 3 and 4 provided real opportunities to deliver corporate university offerings and, by shifting program responsibility to outside vendors, would reduce organizational risk.

Box 11.4
Outlining a
Business Plan
for a Corporate
University:
Starting the
Process

I. Executive Summary
- Concise overview of the business alternatives and their costs
- Description of key details of the planned business alternative, a virtual corporate university, including the required institutional investment and projected development time frame

II. Industry Analysis and Trends
- External environmental analysis
- Trends in organizational development, employee development, and corporate universities
- Consider healthcare and non-healthcare examples

III. Internal Environmental Analysis
- Organizational structure, culture, and environment for the new business

IV. Comparative Analysis
- Comparative analysis (including related financials) for alternative options for a corporate university at Best Health
- Comprehensive discussion of each option, with emphasis on preferred alternative of option 5: virtual corporate university

V. Definition and Description of Virtual Corporate University for Best Health

VI. Operations and Technology Plan for Virtual Corporate University
- Description of how the corporate university would function
- Consideration of technology required, integration with existing technology

VII. Management and Organization for Virtual Corporate University
- Organization and reporting structure for corporate university

VIII. Implementation Plan
- Milestones for program development
- Time frame for program initiation

IX. Evaluation Plan
- Description of short-term and long-term metrics appropriate for university evaluation

X. Financial Statements and Projections
- Supporting financial statements, breakeven analyses, and sensitivity analyses associated with business options
- Specific financials about the virtual corporate university option, supporting plans, and projects

Data from their interviews indicated that outsourcing options had strong advantages: They could be initiated quickly because the curriculum already existed, there would be no need to hire additional Best Health employees, and they could choose a firm that had expertise in healthcare organizations and could also serve as an external consultant. Still, outsourcing had several disadvantages: It could be expensive, its educational programs might not be tailored to the specific needs of Best Health, and it was unlikely to engender senior executive–level ownership of the corporate university learning and development function.

Overall, Green and Miller believed option 5—the virtual model—made the most sense for Best Health. A virtual corporate university could be a "conceptual umbrella" under which Best Health could work to integrate all its current education programs, eventually eliminating redundancy

TABLE 11.1
Benefits and
Costs of a
Corporate
University in
Healthcare

Benefits	Costs
• Consistent approach to curriculum, leadership development • Clearinghouse for many activities, including mandatory clinical education and continuing education • Elimination of redundancies in training and development, thereby reducing costs • Capability to support new initiatives quickly, nimbly • Improved quality of education and training • Comprehensive approach to education: courses that build on each other with common threads and themes (e.g., customer service, patient safety) rather than a collection of unrelated courses • Curriculum directly related to business needs, skill gaps in organization • Shared responsibility for learning	• Staff • Enabling technology —learning management system (either developed in-house or purchased through a vendor) • Classrooms • E-learning modules • Instructors • Materials • Time costs for program participation

and raising program quality. Further, by coordinating all education and training within the virtual corporate university model, Best Health could standardize its leadership messages and save money by eliminating overlapping offerings.

The team met with Long to present the evidence, describe the decision options, and determine next steps. This presentation confirmed their beliefs about option 5 as the most appropriate and viable alternative for Best Health. While Long was intrigued by the outsourcing possibilities of options 3 and 4, she knew she would need senior executives to participate as faculty to solidify their buy-in, and she was reluctant to pursue a program that was not developed in-house. In the end, Long gave the team the green light to develop option 5 into a full-blown business proposal. She emphasized the need to be thorough in their presentation of the evidence and to be as concrete as possible about the financial costs and potential impacts of the various options.

Back in their offices, Green and Miller outlined a business plan that would describe the options for building a corporate university at Best Health and then develop option 5 in detail (Box 11.4), including a list of projected benefits and costs for the initiative (Table 11.1). While they knew costs would be a major concern for the board, they had learned that many

Box 11.5
Three
Implementation
Options for a
Virtual
Corporate
University

Option 5a:
- Hire no additional staff.
- Purchase enabling technology.
- Use internal resources for faculty.
- Charge back education and training costs to units on the basis of use.

Option 5b:
- Develop new curriculum based on organization needs and leadership expectations.
- Purchase enabling technology.
- Use combination of internal and external faculty.

Option 5c:
- Hire education specialists.
- Purchase enabling technology.
- Partner with vendors to develop curriculum, etc.

For any option: Consider phasing in implementation of the corporate university over a multiyear time frame.

of the organization's training and development costs resulted from requirements imposed by the Joint Commission, the Occupational Safety and Health Adminstration, and other regulatory bodies. Thus, a virtual corporate university could help Best Health organize and deliver high-quality education and training to meet these requirements. Once these mandatory costs were taken into account, the additional expenditures for the corporate university could be accounted for incrementally, rather than attributing all education and training to the corporate university.

In addition, Green recognized the value of providing options for implementing a new corporate university (Box 11.5), so she developed a list of potential new programs (Box 11.6) and included them in the business plan. Also, to obtain and maintain executive buy-in for the project, the team recommended creation of a steering committee to further develop and guide implementation of the corporate university. Finally, it developed a formal presentation for Long to use when discussing the corporate university initiative with the Best Health board.

Step 5: The Board Meets and Decides

When Long met with the Best Health board of directors to present her proposal for a new Best Health corporate university, she brought Green and Miller to help make the case. Armed with their evidence and analyses, the presentation was convincing, and the board voted to invest in option

---

Incorporate New Learning Technologies
- New technologies would allow employees to register for courses and take online courses at work or from home.
- Best Health would be able to track participation in mandatory education.

Offer New Development and Training Programs
- A **high-potential program** would be useful to help identify, train, and develop future organizational leaders.
- A **preparation for supervision program** would provide a class for employees to take prior to assuming their first supervisory positions.
- A **mentoring program** would take advantage of outstanding employees at all levels and help them progress in their professional development.

Provide Centralized Learning and Development Opportunities
- Book reviews
- Journal clubs
- Brown-bag lunches
- Executive forums

Box 11.6
New Program Options for a Virtual Corporate University

5—a virtual corporate university for Best Health—with development to begin the following month. However, the board raised several important questions that they insisted be addressed early in program development.

Step 6: Evaluating Results

Board members wanted to make sure data collection mechanisms would be in place to track the program's impact. While they were convinced by the team's needs assessment that a corporate university responded to an important organizational challenge, they also were sensitive to costs. In the absence of immediate and comparable financial information about the value of the project, the board insisted that the team develop an appropriate list of process and outcome metrics, such as return on investment, by which the progress and impact of the project could be monitored and evaluated over time, and then attempt to link them to the Best Health System's balanced scorecard to ensure that the corporate university remained in alignment with the health system's strategic priorities.

Finally, the board was concerned about the linkage between the new virtual entity and existing organizational departments, such as human resources and organizational development. They urged the team to work carefully across organizational boundaries to ensure that the new initiative would have the best chance of success, regardless of existing departmental silos and politics.

Conclusion

Leaving the board meeting, Green and Miller were exhausted but pleased. Their search for evidence had culminated in development of a solid business case that supported an important strategic decision for Best Health. While they knew developing and implementing a virtual corporate university would raise new issues they had not yet considered, they believed their efforts over the previous weeks would help guide the organization through those surprises. And they knew that when the Best Health corporate university was unveiled to employees, they could take pride in their efforts to help Best Health System achieve its vision of being the "best place to work."

Acknowledgments

The author is grateful to Rebecca Schmale, PhD, for her advice and suggestions related to the development of this case and to the editors of this edition who have helped improve this case study. In addition, she is thankful for the financial assistance of the American College of Healthcare Executives (ACHE), which has supported her research on corporate universities in healthcare as part of the 2006 ACHE Health Management Award, and for the targeted assistance of Peter Weil, PhD, FACHE, of ACHE, who provided invaluable insights. Finally, she appreciates the many informants who have participated in her studies of leadership development in healthcare and their contributions to the ideas presented in this case.

TRANSFORMING CEO EVALUATION IN A MULTI-UNIT HEALTHCARE ORGANIZATION

Lawrence Prybil, William Murray, Timothy Cotter, and L. Edward Bryant, Jr.

Introduction

The Sisters of Charity of Leavenworth Health System (SCLHS) is a faith-based, nonprofit healthcare organization. SCLHS sponsors or co-sponsors 11 general-acute hospitals in California, Colorado, Kansas, and Montana. System-wide revenues in fiscal year 2006 were $1.5 billion.

The SCLHS organizational model includes a system-level board of directors, a president and CEO, and corporate staff. Specific responsibilities and decision-making authority are delegated to local boards and CEOs. A system-wide mission statement, core values, and policies unify and provide overall direction for the entire organization.[1]

This chapter describes a transformation of the organization's approach to evaluating the system CEO's performance. It outlines the reasons changes were needed, the principles on which the changes were based, and the evidence-based CEO evaluation model now in place.

Background

In both investor-owned and nonprofit organizations, appointing the CEO, defining his or her performance expectations, and assessing actual performance in relation to those expectations are among the most important duties of a board of directors.[2] National surveys indicate that more than 85 percent of hospital and health system boards now evaluate CEO performance using some type of preset criteria. Similar findings are reported for other types of nonprofit organizations and for investor-owned companies.

However, there are serious questions about the rigor and thoroughness of CEO evaluation processes. Edward Lawler, director of the University of Southern California's Center for Effective Organizations, says that while a majority of companies do evaluate their CEO's performance, "the process is often not very effective because the data they use are provided entirely by the CEO and the internal management system."[3]

153

The CEO performance evaluation system that prevailed at SCLHS during the late 1990s and the early years of the twenty-first century was informal and qualitative. It was a holdover from the system's formative years. In essence, the board chair unilaterally assembled information about the CEO's performance during the past year in relation to objectives previously agreed on by the chair and CEO. The performance measures were not linked directly to the SCLHS incentive compensation program for senior managers, there was minimal input from other board members in the evaluation process, and neither the outcomes of the evaluation process nor the CEO's performance objectives for the coming year were discussed with the board as a whole.

In 2002, L. Edward Bryant, Jr., a senior health attorney at law firm Drinker Biddle, was appointed board chair. This appointment created the opportunity for a fresh look at the CEO performance evaluation and expectation-setting process. This review was timely in view of the 2002 enactment of the Sarbanes-Oxley Act and growing pressures on publicly held and nonprofit organizations for more accountability and better governance.

Designing and Implementing Evidence-Based CEO Evaluation

Step 1: Framing the Issue

The new chair of the SCLHS board; the system CEO, William Murray; and the chair of the board compensation committee, Lawrence Prybil, all recognized the need to modify the approach to setting CEO performance expectations and evaluating the CEO's performance in relation to them. They agreed on the need for a new model that would involve all SCLHS board members (including sponsor representatives), bring better, more quantitative information into the process, and yield written expectations that would provide clear, board-supported guidance for the CEO and, thus, a solid platform for accountability.

This subject was discussed with the board compensation committee and, subsequently, with the board as a whole. As Steve Shortell, dean of the School of Public Health at the University of California–Berkeley, has stated, "The ultimate demand for accountability for the use of the best available information to improve the performance of the organization must come from the board" (Shortell 2006, 26). Both the compensation committee and the board of directors unanimously concurred with the need for a new approach. The compensation committee was charged with designing and implementing a new model and reporting regularly to the entire board.

Steps 2 and 3: Acquiring and Assessing Principles for Evaluation

Applying evidence-based management methods to the issue of CEO performance did not require the committee to seek research-based information (evidence) from many external sources. Rather, in this case, the challenge was to develop a set of principles for system CEO evaluation. The following seven principles, developed by the compensation committee in concert with the system CEO and the committee's independent consultant, Timothy Cotter, became the touchstone.

First, the committee recommended that the SCLHS board annually provide the system CEO with a succinct written list of personal performance objectives on which he or she should place special emphasis during the next year. The objectives should be measurable and linked directly to the SCLHS mission, core values, and strategic plan.

Second, the system CEO and all members of the SCLHS board should have the opportunity to provide input in the process of formulating the CEO's personal performance objectives. The SCLHS board executive committee should adopt these objectives annually and have the flexibility to make modifications or additions during the year if, in its judgment, new opportunities or other circumstances warrant change.

Third, the CEO should be evaluated on demonstrated progress toward achieving the personal performance objectives and on SCLHS operating results in relation to system-wide targets (clinical, financial, etc.) adopted annually by the SCLHS board and included in the dashboard reports provided routinely to the board by SCLHS management. As the person with overall executive responsibility for the system's success, the CEO clearly has accountability for system-wide operating results as well as progress toward the personal performance objectives.

Fourth, the board compensation committee—with technical support provided by an independent consultant and SCLHS staff—should be responsible for coordinating all facets of the evaluation process, including:

- Assembling pertinent information, including the CEO's written self-evaluation, the system's year-end operating performance in relation to targets previously adopted by the board, and input from the SCLHS 360-degree evaluation process, provided by corporate staff and local CEOs;
- Integrating this information into a form that can be sent to all members of the board as a vehicle for obtaining their input and suggestions; and
- Providing the board chair and board executive committee with a comprehensive, unified document for the executive committee to use in completing the CEO evaluation and setting the personal performance objectives for the coming year.

Fifth, the specific steps involved in setting the CEO's performance expectations and evaluation should be codified. To ensure a thorough, expeditious process, responsibility for each of these steps should be assigned and strict timelines for completing them should be delineated.

Sixth, the CEO evaluation process should be based on a fair, objective assessment of the best possible information regarding actual performance in relation to pre-established expectations. The CEO's performance expectations should be linked directly to the SCLHS incentive compensation program, and compensation adjustments should be based on the results of the evaluation process.

Finally, all aspects of the CEO evaluation process should be conducted in a spirit of commitment to continuous improvement—in system-wide operating performance, in the CEO's performance, and in the evaluation process itself. Commitment to evidence-based assessment and ongoing improvement are vital to achieving and maintaining excellence in management and in governance.

Steps 4 and 5: Presenting and Applying the Principles

Based on the seven system-design principles, the committee developed a new evaluation timetable and format, implemented on a pilot basis in 2003. Since this was a brand new process that sought input from all board members, the timetable and format were discussed with the full board before implementation. In response to this input, the board compensation committee and its consultant enabled board members to provide their input regarding the CEO's performance through a secure website.

The overall response to this pilot effort was positive, and the board decided to institutionalize this approach. Based on experience gained in the pilot, certain improvements were made in the process. For example, technical improvements were made to the web-based feedback method, and the timeline was further tightened.

Step 6: Evaluating Results

This new approach to CEO evaluation has been employed for six years (fiscal year 2003 to the present). This method is regularly assessed against the principles described earlier, and refinements have been made every year.

A *process*, of course, is the set of activities a person, group, or organization uses to carry out a particular function. Constant attention to improving core processes is clearly an essential ingredient in achieving organizational success. In this context, there is growing recognition that assessing and improving basic *governance* processes are also key to strengthening board performance. In the case of CEO performance review, the transparency of the process safeguards the integrity of the review and clearly communicates the board's ongoing expectations.

FIGURE 12.1
CEO Evaluation
Process and
Timeline

EXHIBIT A

**SCLHS Chief Executive Officer FY 2006 Performance Evaluation
Process and Timeline**

	Action	Completed By	Date Due
1.	Review draft of CEO evaluation process, form and timeline	Board Compensation Committee with input from the Board Chair	January 10, 2006
2.	Approve final draft of CEO evaluation process, form and timeline	Board Compensation Committee	April 20, 2006
3.	Forward to the Board Chair and Vice Chair results of the CEO's 360 Competency Assessment. CEO submits proposed set of performance objectives for FY 2007	Vice President, Human Resources Chief Executive Officer	June 9, 2006
4.	Add FY 2006 System performance statistics to the CEO evaluation form. (While numbers should be fairly accurate, there could be some audit adjustments as well as a "lag adjustment" on patient satisfaction data.)	Chief Financial Officer SVP, Strategy	July 5, 2006
5.	Forward form with statistics to the Board Chair and Vice Chair	Chief Financial Officer SVP, Strategy	July 6, 2006
6.	Executive Committee meets to: • Determine Executive Committee's assessment of <u>System</u> performance in relation to FY 2006 performance measures • Discuss CEO's proposed performance objectives for FY 2007 • Approve three CEO performance objectives for FY 2007	Executive Committee	July 14, 2006
7.	Submit self-evaluation to Board Chair/Vice Chair	Chief Executive Officer	July 14, 2006
8.	Forward all evaluation materials to Consultant	Vice President, Human Resources	July 24, 2006
9.	Ensure CEO evaluation form contains all required information prior to distribution	Vice President, Human Resources Independent Consultant	July 26, 2006
10.	Distribute CEO performance evaluation form to SCLHS Board members for completion	Independent Consultant	July 31, 2006
11.	Return completed CEO performance evaluation forms to Independent Consultant	Board Members	August 11, 2006
12.	Compile performance evaluation responses from Board members. Prepare and forward long- and short-form summary reports to Board Chair and Vice Chair for review	Independent Consultant	August 23, 2006
13.	Board Chair and Vice Chair, supported by Independent Consultant, finalize short-form summary evaluation report	Board Chair Vice Chair Independent Consultant	August 30, 2006
14.	Distribute short-form summary evaluation report to the Executive Committee (excluding the CEO)	Board Chair Independent Consultant	September 1, 2006 (separate mailing)
15.	Executive Committee meets to: • Discuss CEO performance • Finalize FY 2007 CEO performance objectives • Assist Board Chair to prepare for meeting with - CEO	Executive Committee	September 7-9, 2006 (30-45 minutes during Board Retreat)
16.	Finalize CEO short-form summary evaluation report, including final set of FY 2007 performance objectives and present it to CEO	Board Chair	September 29, 2006
17.	Distribute CEO short-form summary evaluation report to SCLHS Board members in advance of October Board meeting	Independent Consultant	October 4, 2006 (separate mailing)
18.	Review the FY 2006 CEO evaluation process and timeline; identify improvements to make in FY 2007	Board Compensation Committee	October 12, 2006
19.	Review CEO performance report with SCLHS Board	Executive Committee	October 13, 2006

Figure 12.1 indicates the CEO evaluation format used in fiscal year 2006 to integrate:

• system-wide performance targets for fiscal year 2006 and actual operating performance for that period;
• the CEO's self-assessment of performance during fiscal year 2006;
• the collective views of SCLHS board members about the CEO's performance

in relation to the system-wide targets, the personal performance objectives, and the SCLHS leadership competencies for senior executives at the corporate and local level; and

- suggestions offered by board members and the CEO and, when the evaluation process was finished, the CEO's personal performance objectives for fiscal year 2007.

The final steps in the evaluation process included discussion and sign-off by the board executive committee on the completed evaluation form and performance rating and, subsequently, a meeting between the board chair and CEO based on the completed evaluation form. The last step was an executive session of the SCLHS board. At that time, the board chair briefed the board on the content and outcomes of the meeting with the CEO; the board also discussed the evaluation process and ways it could be further improved. Prior to the executive session, the CEO was invited to share his or her perspectives on the evaluation process and outcomes with the board as a whole.

Conclusion

Over the past four years, evaluation of the SCLHS system CEO has been transformed from an informal, noninclusive approach to a model that engages the board as a whole, involves a formalized process with clearly defined steps, and is based on predetermined expectations and objective information regarding actual results in relation to those expectations.

As an integral part of the process, the board compensation committee's independent compensation consultant continually provides current, comparative information regarding compensation practices (including base salary, incentive compensation programs, and benefits) for executives in peer systems throughout the country. The consultant also keeps the committee up to date on pertinent rules, regulations, and reports by government agencies and private organizations. The committee uses this information to ensure that the SCLHS compensation program and practices are fully consistent with contemporary standards, as well as the SCLHS board's compensation philosophy and policy. The committee and its consultant regularly report on these trends and developments to the SCLHS board. The SCLHS board is now well-equipped with information and understanding of executive compensation, which will be helpful in dealing with the Internal Revenue Service's new 990 forms.

The SCLHS board strongly supports this evidence-based approach to providing governance direction for the SCLHS executive compensation program and evaluating the system CEO's performance. All board members are actively engaged in the evaluation process and believe it is fair, is thorough, and meets best-practice standards for nonprofit, tax-exempt organizations.

The system CEO, William Murray, also is fully supportive of the new model and believes it is the most effective evaluation process he has experienced in his career. He has incorporated several elements of this process into setting expectations and evaluating the performance of the local hospital executives. Thus, the SCLHS board's investment of time and effort in improving the system CEO's evaluation process is paying multiple dividends.

There always will be ways to improve the SCLHS approach to CEO evaluation. However, after four years of experience, all parties involved believe this evidence-based model is beneficial for the CEO, the board, and the system as a whole.

Endnotes

1. For information about the system's history, development, and organizational structure, see *Our Common Calling: Sisters of Leavenworth Health System*. Lenexa, KS: Sisters of Charity of Leavenworth Health System, 2006.
2. See, for example, the National Association of Corporate Directors. *Report of the NACD Blue Ribbon Commission on Board Leadership*. Washington, DC: NACD, 2004; Alliance for Advancing Nonprofit Healthcare. *Advancing the Public Accountability of Nonprofit Healthcare Organizations: Guidelines on Governance Practices*, Washington, DC, 2005; and Ryan, W., R. Chait, and B. Taylor. "Problem Boards or Board Problems." *The Nonprofit Quarterly*, Winter 2005, pp. 80–87.
3. "Board Governance and Accountability," an interview with Edward E. Lawler III, conducted by Robert Howie, Jr. Balanced Scorecard Report, Reprint No. B0301D, Harvard Business School Publishing Corporation, 2003, p. 3.

Reference

Shortell, S. 2006. "Promoting Evidence-Based Management." *Frontiers of Health Services Management* 22: 23–29.

IMPROVING PAIN MANAGEMENT IN LONG-TERM CARE

Arthur Webb and Ellen Flaherty

Introduction

Improving quality is often impossible without changing the organization and delivery of services. This case is about a quality improvement initiative to reduce pain in patients requiring long-term care. Examining the case reveals how one shapes the structure and process of an organization to support change and quality.

Village Care of New York is a complex, community-based, not-for-profit urban healthcare organization that provides leadership and innovative services to two underserved populations—older adults and those infected with HIV/AIDS. With our array of programs in SeniorChoices and the Network of AIDS Services, we offer consumer-centered care that promotes independence and respects individual dignity.

In January 2005, we began a quality improvement initiative across 14 different programs. The initiative focused on pain management, a central issue in geriatric and HIV/AIDS care. This initiative became a unifying force for our staff, a catalyst for team spirit, and a focal point of effort.

We served close to 6,000 people in 2006, primarily in Manhattan and Brooklyn. We have been growing at close to 12 percent a year for ten years. Our budget for 2007 is almost $130 million, and we have 1,500 employees.

For nearly 15 years, we has been reshaping our role to be less a provider of specific services and more a patient- or person-centric manager of care across locations, across disciplines, and over time. As much as we are driven by our mission to change services as the needs of those we serve change, translating this mission into practice is daunting at best and troublesome at worst because we are highly dependent on government funding. Government regulations make change an almost insurmountable barrier.

How to build the evidence to demonstrate the value of person-centered care and how to organize services to deliver on this promise are the challenges facing all long-term care providers. Public policy, value aspirations, and goals get organized to deliver on the promise at the provider level, where performance meets the patient. The structure must support quality improvement, not the other way around. Structure does not automatically follow quality goals.

TABLE 13.1
Six Aims for
Quality
Improvement

Care Should Be:

1. *Safe:* Avoid injuries to patients from the care that is intended to help them.
2. *Effective:* Provide services based on scientific knowledge to all who could benefit, and refrain from providing services to those not likely to benefit.
3. *Patient-Centered:* Provide care that is respectful of and responsive to individual patient preferences, needs, and values, and ensure that patient values guide all clinical decisions.
4. *Timely:* Reduce waiting time and sometimes harmful delays for both those who receive and those who give care.
5. *Efficient:* Avoid waste, including waste of equipment, supplies, ideas, and energy.
6. *Equitable:* Provide care that does not vary in quality because of personal characteristics such as gender, ethnicity, geographic location, or socioeconomic status.

SOURCE: Institute of Medicine (2001).

Providers must adopt a construct for quality that is evidence based, results oriented, and accepted by the broader professional and regulatory world as legitimate. Toward this end, the Village Care board adopted the Institute of Medicine's quality framework, outlined in its 2001 report, *Crossing the Quality Chasm,* which focuses on these six domains: safety, timeliness, efficiency, equity, effectiveness, and patient-centeredness (Table 13.1).

The success of the pain management program can be largely attributed to one thing—an integrated team approach. Although the clinical programs were ultimately responsible for actually effecting the change on the front lines, the outcomes would not have been achieved so powerfully without the efforts of many levels of leadership and multiple departments.

Applying Evidence-Based Management

Step 1: Framing the Question

A systematic, step-by-step approach was vital to the success of this initiative (Table 13.2). This overarching question became our touchstone:

Can a quality improvement approach improve utilization of evidence-based pain management strategies across 14 diverse programs?

Key to the initiative's success was the inclusion of pain management in the organization's goals. These goals were set as part of a larger performance management program at Village Care. In the fall of 2006, management

TABLE 13.2
Steps in the Pain
Management
Initiative

1. Arrived at a consensus among senior executives about the importance of pain management and the need for a new approach to organizational improvement.
2. Obtained support from the board of directors to adopt this as a major organizational goal.
3. Assigned top executives to design the program.
4. Established clear goals and an evidence-based approach using a recognized national model.
5. Integrated pain management goals into performance assessment for each program.
6. Established key measures and recording processes.
7. Reviewed and monitored progress at the senior executive level.
8. Reported results to the board of directors.

initiated a comprehensive leadership training program for approximately 120 midlevel managers. Their training included didactic courses and interactive assignments and provided specific tools to facilitate and promote communication and accountability. Managers were expected to use the knowledge and tools gained through this program to achieve measurable results. Their accountability for pain management improvements helped drive the outcomes.

For example, managers were responsible for ensuring that staff job descriptions included language specific to organizational goals (including pain management), translating those goals into expectations, and incorporating those expectations into annual performance reviews.

The success of any initiative depends on establishing goals that are specific and measurable. The goals of the pain initiative, while appearing simplistic and easy to achieve, required multiple layers of change. This change included the integration of evidence-based guidelines and the resultant changes in staff behavior and changes in process and structure of organizational goals (Table 13.3).

The improvement projects varied in their focus. Some examples of these projects are:

- **Village Nursing Home**: *Utilizing a pain data tracking tool to improve the quality and development of interdisciplinary pain care plans.* One interdisciplinary team at Village Nursing Home piloted the use of a tracking tool to help the staff identify residents with pain and develop appropriate care plans.
- **Chelsea and Village Adult Day Centers:** *Engaging staff in the appropriate documentation of pain management through the chart audit process.* Staff at both adult day centers audited all client charts using the Village Care standardized pain chart audit tools and then discussed quality improvement in terms of analysis of their own data.

TABLE 13.3
Performance
Management
Quality Goals

1. Pain Screening
- All programs will assess pain on admission 100% of the time using the seven-question pain screening tool and enter the data into Village Care's electronic database. Sites will pilot the data entry from 1/1/06 until 3/31/06. From 4/1/06 until 6/30/06, pain screening data from all new admissions will be entered into the database. After 7/1/06, all pain screening data completed on admission and routine reassessments will be entered into the database.

2. Client Satisfaction
- All programs will conduct and submit raw data from the client pain satisfaction survey every six months, beginning in February 2006. The participation rate should not be lower than 80% of clients who are cognitively intact and who consent to participate. Programs may alter this schedule according to their client satisfaction survey schedule.

3. Staff Knowledge
- All programs will support the corporate staff satisfaction survey, which will include questions specific to pain knowledge, and will submit raw data every six months in 2006. The participation rate should not be lower than 75% of full-time employees.

4. Process Improvement
- Every six months, all programs will develop at least one improvement project specific to pain, based on the data analysis from their programs. The improvement project should use PDSA (Plan-Do-Study-Act) cycles to implement small tests of change.

- **Treatment Adherence and Case Management:** *Developing a staff education program to improve knowledge and attitudes toward clients with pain.* Using the results of the staff pain knowledge survey, case management and treatment adherence teams helped design an educational program to meet the needs of case managers and health educators.

The nature of the organization and the types of services provided influenced the applicability of information. Initially we adopted a hybrid pain management model based on the nationally recognized work of City of Hope National Medical Center (Duarte, CA) and the University of Wisconsin. In part, the model uses nurse-champions to lead an institutional pain management program. This idea appealed to us because of our organizational diversity and champions' ability to lead organizational change while achieving goals specific to their programs. However, because we did not have nurses for every program, we decided to enlist champions from a wide variety of disciplines and roles. Unfortunately, many of the designated champions were not seen as leaders and were not in a position to hold other individuals accountable. In hindsight, this model was not the best fit for Village Care.

Because of Village Care's decentralized approach to service delivery, we encouraged programs to use the Plan-Do-Study-Act (PDSA) model of small changes. This model allowed each program to fit the pain initiative into its various service offerings with greater ease than a one-size-fits-all approach would have. However, we did demand the same results and information about their initiatives. (Experience with the PDSA method has encouraged innovative approaches to other quality problems, too.)

We were fortunate that the "so what" of this project was so clear that buy-in came easily, especially from frontline staff. The need for change was compelling and communicated frequently to staff at all levels. In addition, the following message to staff linked back to our mission and provided the necessary context for the initiative:

The mistreatment of pain exacts high costs for the individuals who suffer needlessly and for health care institutions that incur higher costs (hospital readmissions, prolonged inpatient stays). The populations cared for by this organization, older adults and people with AIDS, report very high incidences of pain; upwards of 88% of AIDS patients and 86% of older adults experience chronic persistent pain.

Step 2: Acquiring the Evidence

Why did we choose pain from among the many illnesses and frailties confronting the people we serve?

One reason was that a major pain initiative in one of our programs had demonstrated considerable success. We also read many new studies focusing on the undertreatment of pain and its consequences. Two major sources of evidence were our employees—who persistently reported to senior staff that this critical issue was not adequately addressed—and our clients—who repeatedly reminded us that pain was a problem for them. Our clients told us that untreated pain had serious consequences, including the misuse and overuse of pain killers, loss of appetite, and difficulty adhering to treatment regimens. Although pain cannot be verified by medical tests and varies from one patient to another, our emphasis on patient-centeredness obligated us to figure out how to improve this situation.

We began by marshalling an interdisciplinary team, including clinicians and managers from all 14 programs, to lead the initiative. This group, called the Pain Advisory Council (PAC), developed a charter that began with discovery of information:

- We found evidence to demonstrate *need* for improved pain management from:
  - The "voices of our customers"
  - Our mission
  - Published studies demonstrating the undertreatment of pain in older adults and HIV/AIDS clients

- We found that the evidence supporting the *performance management/quality improvement approach* to improving pain management is less robust.
- With respect to the *clinical application* of pain management programs, we found rigorous scientific evidence on assessing and treating pain in both populations.

Our team had to achieve a level of comfort that all the evidence, or lack of it, had been identified and evaluated. This task would have been easier had there been less evidence! Scouring the vast body of literature on how to improve pain management was a challenge. We found it helpful to compare our findings with the thinking of leaders in the field, especially the Institute of Medicine and the Institute for Healthcare Improvement. Knowing that the evidence we had gathered was consistent with what the leaders in the field were saying made us more confident that we were using the best information available to determine our options.

Steps 3 and 4: Assessing and Presenting the Evidence

Early on, we recognized that staff education would be a key component of the pain initiative. The PAC sponsored a two-day educational program to kick off the project. Participants were a diverse group of 75 "champions" selected by their program managers to lead the charge at the grassroots level. This group had a variety of educational backgrounds and roles within the organization, and many struggled to achieve some of the objectives, such as engaging frontline staff in a dialog focused on evaluating evidence.

Similarly, we found that managers varied in their ability to understand and use evidence critically. Most accepted it at face value and did not understand how research design, context, confounding factors, methods, and consistency with other findings affect the applicability of evidence to other (our) situations. Clinical managers related better to clinical research examples and case studies and did not understand the need to consider reliability and validity when using various research tools. For example, managers typically wanted to design their own instruments to gather information from clients or staff, rather than rely on standard, tested instruments.

We had to challenge managers to think about the quality of evidence. We also had to help managers find new evidence where little was available. Case studies collected throughout the project provided persuasive qualitative evidence and let us disseminate best practices throughout the organization.

Ms. E was a homebound, 50-year-old female with multiple chronic illnesses, including HIV/AIDS and recurring opportunistic infections, such as pneumonia, anemia, and severe peripheral neuropathies. Ms. E's non-adherence to her medication regimen was an issue specific to her HIV status and contributed to the pain of her peripheral neuropathies. During one nursing visit, Ms. E reported her pain as an 8 on the 1-to-10 scale. She reported that her pain fluctuated in intensity but was frequently present and had a significant impact on her mobility and appetite. The community health nurse continued to suggest interventions, but Ms. E was reluctant to take pain medications. However, she was receptive to using a newly marketed medication for neuropathy and topical anesthetic patches. She also was receptive to having a social worker visit for short-term counseling. During a follow-up visit two weeks later, Ms. E reported that she had begun using the two new medications and that they had improved her pain to a 4 on the 10-point scale. This improvement prompted her to participate in physical therapy, and she was talking about the possibility of going out to a neighborhood holistic coffee shop. The nurse reported that Ms. E's spirits were uplifted and her overall quality of life improved.

Step 5: Applying the Evidence

The nature of an organization and the types of services it provides influence the applicability of specific information (Damore 2006). As noted, we had to make significant course corrections when our first champion-led strategy was not working well. We should have recognized that big initiatives require custom fitting. Even the best suit requires an experienced tailor to make it look right! We had to determine the factors and information that would help us successfully launch our initiative. Among these factors were the financial and staff resources at hand and the capacity of our managers.

To deliver care in its complex structure, Village Care relies on a delegated model of service delivery, supported by a central core of functional capabilities in human resources, legal, finance, information technology, compliance, marketing, and public relations. Senior executives orchestrate support and guidance. Our respective program managers oversee a wide range of services. Some are responsible for the largest skilled nursing home for AIDS patients in the United States, with a $38 million annual budget; others manage a $2 million community case management program for "hard-to-reach" people living with HIV/AIDS (See Sidebar 13.1).

The same diversity exists in our programs for the elderly. Executives have budgetary and program responsibility for providing high-quality care and achieving the organization's performance goals. They have a wide degree of latitude to establish approaches that best meet the needs of their customers. Although this flexibility often results in unique and innovative solutions, it also produces wide variation in practices throughout Village Care. The pain initiative was an attempt to introduce a new approach to organizational improvement by establishing a standard way of responding to pain.

Another critically important contextual variable was the heightened concern of our board, with respect to quality of care and accountability. Board members asked a simple but powerful question: How do we know that quality is being delivered at the patient level? The board and senior executives agreed that we would use the pain initiative as the beginning step in answering this question.

This initiative would not only improve pain management but serve as an internal model for improvements on other quality indicators. It would help us learn to make improvements effectively, measure and report on change, and efficiently integrate organizational improvements system-wide. These organization goals, established under our performance management (PM) structure, facilitated the successful outcome of the pain program at Village Care. Most important, the PM program promoted accountability across various programs.

One daunting challenge was measuring and tracking outcomes efficiently across 14 programs. Over time we concluded that an electronic medical record (EMR) would be a necessary tool to facilitate quality improvement in general and specifically in the pain management project. As a result, Village Care is currently tackling another ambitious goal— development and implementation of an EMR system that embraces quality as the central outcome. We could not have set this transforming goal without first engaging in the pain quality improvement project. Successfuly implementing an EMR system requires the use of nationally accepted and valid protocols of care, reengineered workflow processes, extensive staff training, and development of new leadership capacity. The pain initiative gave us the opportunity to practice all these skills.

Conclusion

In 2005, Village Care of New York embarked on a process to achieve an audacious goal: transforming the organization by integrating quality improvement strategies, using improvements in pain management as a model. Several key lessons emerged:

- The success of any initiative to improve quality of care must begin with the patient. The change of

Sidebar 13.1 SeniorChoices and the Network of AIDS Services

SeniorChoices includes:
- Village Nursing Home, a 200-bed skilled nursing facility specializing in short-term rehabilitation;
- two adult day health programs serving 100 people;
- a large community information and referral program reaching close to 1,500 people;
- a senior housing project with services for 100; and
- a care advocate program that helps seniors in organized services.

The Network of AIDS Services includes:
- Rivington House, a 200-bed skilled nursing center for AIDS patients only;
- two medical day programs;
- a diagnostic and treatment center;
- three home care models, including a large certified home health agency, a licensed home care agency providing paraprofessional services, and a specialized long-term home health program;
- a case management program;
- a specialized medication management program; and
- a community resource center in Brooklyn's Red Hook neighborhood.

behavior at the bedside depends on significant buy-in from the clinical team. In the case of pain management, the overall goals of the initiative made sense at every level.

- Keep the goals simple. The goal of screening every new admission for pain 100 percent of the time was simple, yet it paved the way for integrating the concepts of evidence-based management into the fabric of the organization. Our PM program reinforced the need for measuring outcomes and establishing accountability.
- Converting the acquisition of new knowledge into behavior change occurs at a snail's pace. While it may take only a short time for staff to understand the concepts, widespread application of the requisite skills is accomplished over the long haul, with persistent practice and mentoring.

These lessons provide Village Care with sound guidance for future action. As healthcare reimbursement methods move toward pay-for-performance models and value-based purchasing, our organization has recognized that using the concepts and skills of evidence-based management will help us meet the challenges ahead.

References

Damore, J. 2006. "Making Evidence-Based Management Usable in Practice." *Frontiers of Health Services Management* 22: 41–44.

Institute of Medicine. 2001. *Crossing the Quality Chasm: A New Health System for the 21st Century.* Washington, DC: National Academies Press.

14

THE BUSINESS CASE FOR A HOSPITAL PALLIATIVE CARE UNIT: JUSTIFYING ITS CONTINUED EXISTENCE

Kenneth R. White and J. Brian Cassel

Introduction

New healthcare services and products generally are presented to management first through a business plan. Successful plans undergo an organizational approval process that culminates in their adoption. Business plan preparation is taught in business schools, and the approval process is well understood. What is not routine is the formal evaluation of the new service or product *after* implementation, to determine whether experience correlates with the assumptions and projections in the initial plan and whether the service or product warrants continuation. In other words, *does the evidence support the initial decision to implement the service or product?* This case presents such an opportunity: the evaluation of an existing service to justify its continued existence, in terms of patient outcomes and financial impact.

This case is based on the late 2002 experience of a large, southeastern academic medical center, part of a large health sciences campus with schools of medicine, dentistry, pharmacy, nursing, and allied health. In fiscal year 2003, the medical center had 779 licensed beds (681 of which were staffed), 30,336 inpatient admissions, 179,854 inpatient days, and 530,270 outpatient visits. The organization had a traditional functional reporting structure and standard clinical service lines, and its medical staff was also the faculty for the medical school.

Oncology was a particularly strong service line, and the oncology department was a nationally recognized leader in training programs and patient outcomes. Oncology included a 30-bed medical-surgical unit, a separate bone marrow and stem cell transplant unit (13 beds), and several clinics on the main campus and in suburban satellite locations. From this base, clinical staff proposed adding a new palliative care unit.

What Is Palliative Care?

People with end-of-life conditions[1] have a choice in the kind of care they receive. They may want aggressive care, even if the prospects for improvement are slim, or they may choose palliative care—that is, services geared not to "cure" but rather to provide comfort, including pain control, in a holistic manner. It involves not just the relief of physical symptoms, but also attention to the emotional and spiritual needs of patients and families.

Palliative care is both a medical specialty and an approach to care for patients with advanced, chronic, or life-limiting illnesses or injuries. It is not only for those in the final days and weeks of life, but a choice that is made between the patient and the physician to forgo more costly, highly technical interventions intended to prolong life.

Although an increasing number of hospitals offer palliative care services, many patients and families do not know such services exist, they may have misconceptions about them, or their physicians may not recommend them for various reasons. Hospital-based palliative care usually involves an interdisciplinary team of providers, including a clinical leader (palliative care physician or advanced practice nurse), counselors, psychologists, clergy, social workers, physical therapists, and a dedicated nursing staff trained in caring for patients with life-limiting illnesses. Palliative care can be provided on an inpatient basis through hospital consultative services or in designated units, or on an outpatient basis by hospital staff or under the auspices of a hospice. (Hospices provide many palliative care services, usually in an individual's home, and have a well-established organizational model and philosophy.)

In the late twentieth century and into the early twenty-first century, the palliative care movement gained momentum as a patient care approach. In 2003, more than 1,025 hospitals had formal palliative care programs, and between 2000 and 2005, the number of such programs grew 96 percent. With this rapid diffusion of innovation, hospital-based palliative care programs were beginning to show an impact on clinical and nonclinical outcomes.

Palliative Care in Our Medical Center

Recognizing the U.S. trend toward improving end-of-life care and pain management, the physicians of this medical center were early champions of palliative care and received grants and contracts to study ways to improve the care of people with life-limiting illnesses. Even before developing a specialized palliative care unit, medical center management was committed to providing a consultative end-of-life care and pain management service, initially with patients in the oncology center.

Between 1994 and 1997, the chair of the oncology department was instrumental in receiving approval for a dedicated palliative care unit from the medical center's administration. Using two internal quality improvement studies, the physician and the pain management specialist documented significant unmet end-of-life needs and the occurrence of futile care in the hospital.[2] The goals of the initial proposal were to improve care for patients with life-limiting illnesses and conditions, to develop a team of professionals to deliver the most appropriate care to those who chose to forgo life-prolonging treatments, and to alleviate pain and suffering for patients and their families. As part of an academic medical center, the hospital's other goals for the program included research, teaching, training, and potential cost savings.

During this time, the physician champion had developed a team of professionals who were specially trained in end-of-life care: nurses, a pain management specialist, chaplains, social workers, and others. Although the medical center provided end-of-life consultation services and was affiliated with community hospice organizations, it did not offer a formal, dedicated palliative care service until approval was granted in 1997.

Over the following 30 months, the physician and nurse champions were able to garner external funding to establish the new unit. Two physicians and the pain management specialist were selected as Project on Death in America scholars; the Jessie Ball du Pont Foundation provided almost $300,000; and the local Thomas Hospice Foundation provided another $100,000 in funds, plus contributions of labor and materials used to renovate the space. In combination with the internal data demonstrating the clinical need for this new program, these funds made a compelling financial case for program feasibility.[3]

The unit opened in May 2000 with 11 beds, 11.3 full-time equivalent nurses (including a pain management specialist), and part-time staff from many other departments as needed—social work, chaplaincy, pharmacy, occupational therapy, physical therapy, and others. The decision to create a dedicated unit, rather than the more common consultative service with no dedicated beds, was critical, and it became the crux of the arguments surrounding the program's continued existence.

The palliative care team was convinced that a dedicated unit would better achieve its clinical, training, and research goals than would a purely consultative service. Clinically, the team hoped that a different kind of acute inpatient environment—quieter, more homelike, available to family visitors 24/7—would be comfortable and attractive to patients and families. This environment could be a tangible way to show patients and families that palliative care was not synonymous with "doing less," but rather a choice to "care more."

A second reason a dedicated unit might improve clinical outcomes was that its staff of dedicated, experienced nurses and physicians would be spending most of their time with patients having similar needs for symptom management and end-of-life care. The team wanted to create a setting where 90 percent or more of patients needed palliative care, since earlier research in oncology and other fields had shown that high-volume specialist care produces better clinical and financial outcomes than low-volume care.

A third way in which the team believed a dedicated unit would result in better clinical outcomes was through clinical control. In most palliative care consultation programs, the consultants make recommendations to the attending physician, who may ignore or modify the advice. A dedicated unit would allow the team to establish its own clinical algorithms and monitor the implementation of best practices. Finally, patients could be admitted directly to the dedicated unit from the emergency department.

After nearly two years of operation, the team's optimism appeared to have been well-placed. The unit was deemed successful in terms of clinical outcomes and patient, family, and physician satisfaction. Utilization and outcome data showed an average daily census of five to seven patients (55 to 77 percent of capacity) and a growing number of referrals from oncologists and other physician specialists. The number of medical center patients transferred to the unit from intensive care also had increased.

But would positive clinical outcomes be sufficient to sustain the unit as financial pressures on the hospital increased? The answer, we learned, was "maybe not."

Applying Evidence-Based Management

Step 1: Formulating the Research Question

In 2002, our medical center, like many others in an increasingly cash-strapped era, contracted with a consulting group to improve overall hospital efficiency and find ways to decrease costs without compromising quality. The consulting group's initial analysis of the cost-effectiveness of various hospital services and units was based on the service to which patients were assigned (for example, medical, surgical, cardiac) or hospital unit (intensive care, nursing, palliative care) *at the time of discharge*. The consulting group simply compared the total reimbursement generated by a service/unit to its total cost to determine cost-effectiveness.

This methodology led the consultants to conclude that the palliative care unit was not financially viable: Costs for patients discharged from the palliative care unit significantly exceeded reimbursement for their care. They recommended the unit be closed. In fact, they placed it at the top of their list of recommended cuts and closures. Outcomes such as documented improvements in quality, symptom management, and patient satisfaction did not outweigh the consultants' concerns over the financial metrics, when the institution's financial survival was at stake.

Thus, the palliative care team's research question became: *How do we "retell the financial story" of the palliative care unit through new analytic methods?*

Step 2: Acquiring Information

The palliative care program staff had to develop a credible challenge to the consultants' financial analysis. We could not respond merely with "finances are unimportant" or "our oncology program needs comprehensive supportive care, symptom management, and end-of-life care as part of its offerings" or "we need a base for our research in these areas." Just as start-up grants were a necessary part of the case for starting the program, the team would have to demonstrate a positive financial contribution to the hospital for the unit to continue.

Unfortunately, we found little in the published literature on the financial contributions of hospital-based palliative care programs. There were a few articles from a program at the Cleveland Clinic, which indicated that no palliative care unit could be financially viable unless its average daily census was 70 to 80 percent of capacity (Davis et al. 2001). This information helped the program determine a possible solution to one aspect of the unit's high costs and low reimbursements: increase the number of palliative care patients, or open the unit to "overflow" patients from oncology and general medicine. The hospital asked the program to do both.

Lacking additional guidance from the literature, the program turned to the newly formed Center to Advance Palliative Care (CAPC) at Mount Sinai Medical School in New York City. Staff there recommended two advisors to help the team, and their engagement with us was funded by a grant from the Robert Wood Johnson Foundation.[4] CAPC and the foundation saw a critical opportunity for the field: The financial case for hospital-based palliative care needed to be greatly strengthened or the movement would fail. If our advisers could convince the hospital's consulting firm that palliative care produced a positive financial outcome, other palliative programs could, too. What could not have been predicted then was how the results of our advisers' work would become a benchmark for measuring the financial contributions of palliative care programs nationwide.

Our palliative care program had one significant advantage: It was organizationally situated in the oncology service line, which had a dedicated financial analyst who had access to all the necessary data sources that we and our advisers would need to paint our financial picture.

Steps 3 and 4: Assessing and Presenting the Evidence

We and our advisers saw the first ray of light when we recognized that the consulting firm's conclusion that the costs of caring for palliative care patients significantly exceeded reimbursement was based on a faulty assumption. Because the palliative care program was the last to "touch" these patients, the consultants assigned the costs of patients' entire admission to the unit. (Recall that the consulting group performed its financial evaluations using the service or unit *at discharge*.) With this analytic method, a unit-based program (in contrast to a consultation program model) inevitably appears on paper to incur high costs, relative to reimbursement.

The team needed to show the consulting group that the dedicated palliative care unit brought together patients who were among the most complicated, complex, gravely ill individuals served by the hospital and who often had already been at the hospital for a long time before they arrived on the palliative care unit. Hospital data revealed that about half of the palliative care patients had received care on other inpatient units, where the vast majority of their costs were incurred. On average, they did not transfer to the unit until they had been hospitalized more than ten days. By the time many of them were transferred to the palliative care unit, the costs of their care had *already* exceeded the eventual reimbursement. Clarifying this situation was the first step in the team's response to the consulting group.

The second step was to show that, following the transfer to palliative care, costs were significantly lower than those incurred for previous clinical services on other units. The financial analyst disaggregated the costs of individual admissions to show this difference, day by day. This part of the analysis showed that transferring patients to palliative care actually saved several hundred thousand dollars in costs *per patient*.

The third step was to extend this argument with a "what if" analysis. This premise proposed that if more of the hospital's terminally ill patients had been transferred to the palliative care unit—even after spending two weeks in conventional treatment units—the hospital would have saved several hundred thousand *additional* dollars in costs annually for these patients' remaining days in the hospital.

The evidence from our assessment that the hospital's consulting group found most compelling was a simple table of three-year data on the 224 adults aged 65 or older who died in the hospital after a stay of at least 14 days. The table compared their average cost per day (about $2,500) to the average cost per day for patients on the palliative care unit (about $1,000). The analysis determined that had all of these patients transferred to the palliative care unit on the 15th day of their hospitalization and spent their remaining inpatient days (averaging 20) there, the medical center would have saved more than $6.4 million. (Removing indirect costs from this calculation—for example, social services, medical records, utilities, and hospital administration—would have lowered this figure to about $3.2 million.)[5]

To increase the number of patients served by the palliative care unit, the team asked attending physicians to explain the palliative care option to suitable patients and encourage transfers to the palliative care unit, when appropriate. Physician groups were informed about the unit and the types of patients and families who might benefit from it.

Since about half of the unit's patients were admitted directly to it, these patients' costs and reimbursement were analyzed separately. In these cases, the consulting firm's assumption that the palliative care unit was responsible for all of their costs was correct. Contrary to what we expected, our analysts found that in general these patients' costs also exceeded the reimbursement. We determined that this excess was caused by an unexpectedly high volume of patients admitted under contracts with local hospices. For these patients, the medical center could be reimbursed only the hospice per diem rate for acute care, which is considerably lower than the hospital's normal per diem rate. By contrast, directly admitted patients were profitable. The consulting group recommended that these contracts be renegotiated or terminated. (When renegotiation proved impossible, the contracts were terminated the following year.)

Step 5: Applying the Evidence to the Decision

Our alternative methods of analyzing the palliative care unit's costs and reimbursements convinced the consulting group and hospital management that the unit provided a financial benefit to the hospital. As a result, they approved the unit's continued operation, on the condition that the palliative care team take three steps:

1. Increase its census to reduce daily costs per patient;
2. Renegotiate or terminate the hospice contracts; and
3. Increase referrals, especially from the hospital's intensive care units (which were at their physical capacity and which had the highest costs per day of any unit in the hospital).

In this case study, the palliative care analysts and the consulting firm used the same cost data generated by the hospital's computerized cost-accounting system but came to different conclusions. Novel aspects of the analysis that required conceptual buy-in were: (1) the disaggregation of the entire admission into discrete portions and days and (2) the "what if" scenarios that demonstrated that comfort care and its consequent cost avoidance were not occurring naturally in the hospital without the intervention of the palliative care team. Acceptance of these analyses led to the conclusion that much more could—and should—be done to bring palliative care to appropriate patients.

Ongoing Analysis

Despite the positive conclusion of our presentations to management and their consultants, we did not want to rest on our analytic laurels. More recently, we have used a variety of data (not just related to cost avoidance) to make the case that the palliative care team should be increased in size by adding another full-time advanced practice nurse and a portion of a physician position.

The program has gone on to document its clinical and quality outcomes and has won national and international awards and additional state and national grants to promulgate palliative care. Although survival forced us to conduct a thoughtful review of the unit's financial performance, the palliative care team's perspective is that the unit's most important outcome is greatly improved clinical care and quality of life for patients and families.

Applicability to Consultative Service-Only Models

Since most hospital-based palliative care programs offer consultative services only (no dedicated beds or specialized units), to what extent do our findings apply to them? In the last few years, consultative programs have demonstrated cost avoidance patterns similar to those of programs with dedicated units. In fact, the cost of care in such programs can be quite low, since the physician consultations are reimbursable, and the costs of advanced practice or palliative care nurses' consultations and other team members' time are usually modest. Start-up costs for consultation-only programs are low, if indeed they have any costs other than personnel, whereas start-up costs for a dedicated unit can be significant, although they may be offset by start-up grants or philanthropy.

Step 6: Evaluating Results

Through this analytic process, we learned that three strong variables affect the financial sustainability of palliative care programs:

1. Physicians who perform inpatient consultations or outpatient visits can usually be reimbursed, thus covering their own time.
2. Reimbursement for patients admitted directly into palliative care must be part of the financial analysis, and since we terminated our hospice contracts, our reimbursement for such patients has modestly exceeded costs each year for the past four years. This margin is sensitive to patients' length of stay.
3. Most cost avoidance analyses for patients transferred into palliative care from other services/units assume that reimbursement is unaffected because the lion's share of reimbursement is from fixed-payment payers, such as Medicare. With fixed reimbursements, the financial benefit of palliative care derives almost solely from its lower costs. (DRG-exempt hospitals [i.e., hospitals that are reimbursed based on costs rather than diagnosis-related groups], such as those in Maryland or cancer hospitals, may have to pursue a different kind of analysis.)

One of the key factors in the success of this program evaluation was the involvement of the financial analyst, who worked closely with the palliative care team. The analyst came to understand the nature of the program and its operational and financial implications, and in turn, the clinical team came to understand the financial implications of its policies and practices.

Broader Applicability of Our Methods

Other palliative care programs trying to make a business case for their operations and wanting to apply our analytic approach need reliable cost data from their home institutions and a financial analyst willing to understand the operations of the palliative care unit and analyze the cost data appropriately. In fact, having a financial analyst familiar with palliative care has become such a clear need that the CAPC's Palliative Care Leadership Center training program offers a discount to hospital teams that include an analyst.[6] This nationwide training program incorporates the analytic methods described in this case, which also have been published (White et al. 2006).

New programs, which are making projections about the potential impact of a service that does not yet exist, also will find online tools and training programs based on our experience—and that of many other programs—through the CAPC.

The most difficult aspects of making financial projections for palliative care are determining which patients would have been appropriate for the service and which of them would actually have been referred for a consult or transferred to a palliative care unit. Despite the variation in hospital organizations and a parallel diversity in palliative care programs, once engaged, they consistently demonstrate a savings of 14 to 40 percent or more in direct or variable costs for the last three to six days of patients' admissions.

Endnotes

1. An end-of-life condition is one that that will cause death, either imminently or at some time in the foreseeable future.
2. "Futile care" is cure-oriented treatment intended to prolong life, despite deterioration of the patient's condition past the point where the treatment will be of benefit. Worse, futile care often causes unnecessary suffering and side effects. And, since it often takes place in intensive care settings, it can be costly.
3. For more information on the history of this and other such programs in the United States, see "Pioneer Programs in Palliative Care: Nine Case Studies" at www.milbank.org/reports/pppc/0011pppc.html.
4. For more information on this engagement from the perspective of the external advisors, see "Two Struggling Academic Palliative Care Centers

Get Management Advice to Help Stabilize" at www.rwjf.org /reports/grr/046742.htm.

5. In 2002, the palliative care team had not yet refined its analyses to the point of removing indirect costs, which accrue regardless of unit. Subsequently, the team was able to calculate only direct costs in estimating cost savings. Cost data were produced by the hospital's cost accounting department. Charge and reimbursement data were provided by the hospital's decision support department via the Massey Cancer Center Information System.

6. See www.capc.org/palliative-care-leadership-initiative.

References

Davis, M. P., D. Walsh, K. Nelson, D. Konrad, and S. B. LeGrand. 2001. "The Business of Palliative Medicine: Management Metrics for an Acute-Care Inpatient Unit." *American Journal of Hospice and Palliative Care* 18: 26–29.

White, K. R., K. G. Stover, J. B. Cassel, and T. J. Smith. 2006. "Non-Clinical Outcomes of Hospital-Based Palliative Care." *Journal of Healthcare Management* 51: 253–67.

USING EVIDENCE IN INTEGRATED CHRONIC CARE MANAGEMENT

Kyle L. Grazier

Background

Depression causes massive personal and societal costs. By 2020, depression is predicted to be the world's second most common disease, responsible for 15 percent of the disease burden worldwide (Lopez et al. 2006). The National Comorbidity Study and other U.S.-based research estimate the point prevalence of depression in the United States at 5 to 14 percent (Kessler et al. 2005). Depression is recognized for its chronicity and its disease burden—and for its responsiveness to treatment. In fact, most clinicians believe that with case finding and managed treatment, much of the pain, suffering, and cost of this condition could be reduced.

Many adults with depression don't seek care, but when they do, the majority seek treatment from their primary care practitioner rather than a mental health specialist. Unfortunately, most primary care practices are not equipped with the clinical expertise, information systems, workflow techniques, and other evidence-based management tools and systems necessary to provide appropriate care for this chronic illness.

Applying Evidence-Based Management

Step 1: Formulating the Research Question

This case describes the development, implementation, and evaluation of a chronic care management model of depression treatment within primary care group practices associated with a major midwestern academic medical center. The story will illustrate how EB management principles and practices apply to the structure of the resultant delivery model, the change processes required, and the model's acceptance by managers, providers, and patients. Put simply, the question for us was, *How can we integrate the best approach to depression treatment within primary care?* We decided to design a model approach based on the best clinical and organizational evidence and then assess its effectiveness through a case-control study.

Step 2: Acquiring the Evidence

Clinical Research on Effectiveness of Treatment

Although the specific procedures, therapies, and medicines have changed rapidly over the past decade, diagnostic classifications and treatment of depression have existed for more than a half century. Applied research into the effectiveness of treatment, however, is much more recent. Few large-scale trials have demonstrated long-term outcomes for various treatments across the range of illness severity and clinical specificity. Instead, research has focused on individual illnesses or categories of illnesses, such as schizophrenia or bipolar disorders. This focus allows researchers to isolate the factors correlated with the individual, the nature of the disease, and the duration of treatment.

Research done in the early 1990s demonstrated the relationships among social, cognitive, and work function characteristics of patients and the outcomes of different types of treatment for major depressive disorders. For almost 50 years, three forms of therapy have dominated depression treatment: psychotherapy, pharmacotherapies, and electroconvulsive therapies. Since more has become understood about the natural history and chronicity of depression, these treatments are often combined at different points in the course of treatment.

In most clinical fields, including depression management, cost-effectiveness and efficacy trials continue to inform best practices. For example, one consequence of an efficacy trial on the use of pharmacotherapy for depression was the key realization that, with proper use of validated screening tools and clear algorithms for choice and dose of medication, depression could be treated in an outpatient setting, and by clinicians who are not mental health specialists—namely, primary care providers.

Research also showed that adults with symptoms of depression were presenting frequently in family practice and primary care physicians' offices. Often, the illness was not recognized and masked as complaints of physical ailments. If the illness were recognized, providers referred patients to mental health specialty clinics (if insured) or community mental health centers (if not insured), or treated the patients themselves. There were no widely available, validated screening tools with which to assess the risk, presence, or severity of depression, or to differentiate depression from other disorders.

Grant support provided the opportunity to test several management mechanisms to improve within primary care settings the quality of the recognition, treatment, and follow-up of people with depression.

Delivery System Management Research on Collaborative Primary Care and Specialty Mental Health Models

At the initiation of this experiment, there was little in the published literature on integration of depression and primary care, or more broadly on collaborative care models for specialty mental health care and primary care delivery. There were, however, research findings from continuing and chronic care models tested for diabetes, heart disease, HIV/AIDS, and asthma. Given the recent recognition of depression as a chronic disease, management research from the chronic disease literature could help us choose models and methods.

Some of the most promising strategies rely on "integration" of physical and mental health services to overcome past problems with financing, purchasing, and delivery of care. "Integration" has a variety of interpretations. Some integrated programs are relatively simple efforts to improve communication and coordinate care; others require the co-location and full engagement of physicians and mental health professionals. The most complex integration strategies include housing, transportation, income support, and mental health and addiction services. Some state initiatives help families and providers identify children with developmental problems and help families find resources and connect with service programs. Still, successful models of integrated psychiatric and medical care within physician practices remained rare.

Evident from most of the literature was the need for a carefully conceived infrastructure to support integrated services. These components were not only physical—such as computer-based information systems—but also cultural. Organizations have unique characteristics—power structures, capacities for change, personnel mix, leadership, and client-provider relationships—that are part of their infrastructure.

Examining the literature on organizations informed the types of processes and mechanisms we would use to define and evaluate our intervention—the bundle of services we would implement in the case practices but not in the control practices. We also would monitor processes and outcomes before and after implementation to gauge the nature and extent of any changes. Evidence from studies of other chronic illnesses indicated that the following components of management models should be considered for our research:

- Identification of champions for the intervention in the clinics
- Extensive education of providers and staff
- An electronic data system that would support a patient registry
- Shared medical and mental health information, communication among sites and practitioners, and documented clinical outcomes
- The capture of direct and indirect costs associated with the care and the intervention

Economic research indicates that financial incentives help promote behavior change. Recognizing these incentives was important in designing our intervention, because in busy primary care clinics, clinicians might not be easily persuaded to add more time to a medical visit so that depression could be assessed or treated. In most cases, this time would not be reimbursed without an appropriate procedure and billing code, neither of which existed.

The literature on the power of non-financial incentives to encourage, reward, or punish behavior is equally compelling. Recent research on primary care practice indicates that physician satisfaction is generally low; many complaints emanate from the breadth of patient conditions seen and lack of access to the specialist expertise needed to treat them effectively. Primary care physicians are responsible for knowing an overwhelming number of clinical guidelines and best practices. By enabling them to quickly consult the clinical information or the mental health specialist for treatment advice or referral, physicians gain confidence in their ability to effectively treat the more complex cases of depression that appear in their caseloads.

Step 3: Assessing the Validity, Quality, and Applicability of the Evidence

The underlying goal of the study was to determine whether and how depression care can be delivered to more individuals at their points of entry into the healthcare system. In addition, we needed an assessment of satisfaction of providers, staff, and patients and a longitudinal measure of change processes. Finally, the proposed processes had to be financially sustainable for the providers, clients, and payers.

To test the feasibility and sustainability of the integration of primary care and depression treatment, we implemented a pre-post, case-control design in natural settings. We applied an intervention—a bundle of processes—to the cases but not to the controls. Data were collected on key measures one year prior to study initiation and throughout the following two years.

Fifteen primary care practices in a three-county area participated, all of which were part of a university faculty group practice plan. Eight case sites received extensive training in the screening, coding, scheduling, and treatment of depression. If patients screened positive for depression, their physicians offered them the opportunity to participate in the study. If they consented (in writing), their information was added to the registry. Participating patients received telephone calls from advanced practice psychiatric nurses, who conducted health assessments, offered advice, and planned follow-up visits to the mental health specialist or primary care provider. The case manager determined the number and time between calls upon assessment of case severity and the patterns of response to medication and other treatment. Control sites conducted business as usual.

To measure clinical outcomes, patients were assessed in person, using the PHQ-8 or PHQ-9 (Patient Health Questionnaire, version 8 or 9) depression assessment instrument, and by phone. The PHQ scores were entered into the shared medical record so that primary care and specialty mental health practitioners could assess patients' most recent health status, examine patterns in the depression symptoms, and modify treatment if necessary. Patients also had access to a printout of their PHQ scores over time.

Surveys and focus groups conducted at several points in the study measured the satisfaction of patients, providers, nurse case managers, and clinic staff.

The study included several mechanisms to determine the economic consequences of the intervention. In an effort to understand portions of the intervention's total costs, we conducted a time and motion study of care managers to determine the direct costs, and later the indirect costs, of their activities. Randomly drawn days and times were selected, during which project staff recorded what they were doing and how long it took. These data were translated into costs using wage, benefit, space, and material charges. Financial managers at the primary care practice sites provided detailed indirect costs of facilities used in the treatment of patients and direct costs of labor and materials.

The second economic objective was to sustain the integrated care program through third-party payment. A new procedure code was created and registered so that billing offices could assign a charge to the resources consumed in the delivery of consultation, therapy, or medication management. We analyzed three years of health plan claim records to capture characteristics of the patients, services, and costs associated with the integrated services and all other services.

No one has ever said that redesigning healthcare systems would be easy. The organizations, in this case the primary care practice sites, enrolled subjects and screened clients earlier and more efficiently when there was a "champion" on-site to educate, promote the concept, and be a resource for questions. If an internal champion did not exist, substantial success was nevertheless attained if the study research coordinator or the nurse case managers frequently visited the site.

The registry began as a stand-alone database but was slowly incorporated into the online electronic medical record system. Computer-based and accessible patient assessments and medication records enabled more timely follow-up calls and more communication between mental health specialty providers and primary care practices.

Satisfaction, as measured by questionnaires, was high among all participants in the study, particularly physicians. The primary care physicians were not motivated by the financial incentives; they wanted to deliver the appropriate therapies, without regard for remuneration. For them, the greatest utility came from having an easy way to access the mental health specialist or to assign a case manager. They also reported that the new system gave them confidence that they were doing the right thing.

Step 4: Presenting the Evidence

Sustaining the project beyond grant funding was one of our biggest challenges. To persuade employers to support benefits packages that would include integrated services, we needed to make a business case for the value of the investment. Convincing benefits officers and financial managers of the value of this approach took considerable time and a level of evidence that the study could not fully support. The returns on investment required by employers were difficult to calculate, given what we did *not* measure, such as gains in productivity or reductions in future acute or emergency care expenses. While the improvements in the clinical depression scores among case subjects were noteworthy, the study could not directly translate them into cost savings for employers.

Step 5: Applying the Evidence in Decision Making

The depression and primary care case described above illustrates the importance of understanding organizational culture, process and outcome evaluations, cost accounting, and shared decision making, as well as the need to make both a clinical and financial case for changing the care delivery and payment systems.

Much of the managerial infrastructure built for the study remains, as does the clinical information system, the case management operations (although they are now part of a broader clinical case management department), and depression screening systems at all clinics. An electronic clinical information tracking system allows primary care providers to communicate with or view communications among different providers concerning a particular patient.

The business case—the evidence that integration is worth its additional cost—is still being generated. Efforts at several large local employers are under way to implement and pay for a depression care management system based on this integration study. Despite the dearth of gold-standard randomized controlled trials, there is sufficient practice-based evidence that care for people with depression can improve by expediting communication of critical information among patients, providers, and payers. The essence of the evidence generated here has been applied to clinical decision making by clinicians, organizations, and patients. Medical practices in other communities are replicating and evaluating these methods. Perhaps the highest form of application of evidence to decision making is efforts like these, which attempt to coordinate better the care of the person, not merely the individual illness.

References

Kessler, R. C., W. T. Chiu, O. Demler, K. R. Merikangas, and E. E. Walters. 2005. "Prevalence, Severity, and Comorbidity of 12-Month DSM-IV Disorders in the National Comorbidity Survey Replication." *Archives of General Psychiatry* 62 (6): 617–27.

Lopez, A. D., C. D. Mathers, M. Ezzati, D. T. Jamison, and C. J. Murray. 2006. "Global and Regional Burden of Disease and Risk Factors, 2001: Systematic Analysis of Population Health Data." *Lancet* 367 (9524): 1747–57.

DATA-DRIVEN INPATIENT BED PLANNING

Jancy Strauman

Background

In the early 1990s many experts predicted that managed care and less invasive procedures would greatly reduce the need for hospital inpatient beds. Hospitals responded by shifting capital investments to ambulatory care and off-site locations and converting double-occupancy rooms to singles. These bed-need predictions failed to consider critical factors, such as the aging of the American population, the influx of younger immigrants, and the closing of some hospitals due to financial challenges. Many hospitals now continually operate with greater than 85 percent utilization—technically "full"— which results in difficulty in scheduling procedures, emergency department diversions, and other operational snags.

The following case study shows how Acme Medical Center, a large quaternary academic medical center located in an urban environment, evaluated and realigned its inpatient beds to better meet current and future needs. During the study period, fall 2004 to spring 2005, Acme operated 698 inpatient beds housed in four inpatient towers. The bed complement included 472 adult medical and surgical beds (168 surgical general care, 188 medical general care, 32 neuroscience general care, and 84 critical care). The pediatric service included 76 general care beds, 14 critical care beds, and 48 beds in the neonatal intensive care unit (NICU). In addition, the hospital had 46 obstetrical and 42 psychiatric beds. By and large, these beds were full; Acme averaged 86 percent utilization during the 18 months prior to the realignment. In addition, it was implementing a strategic plan that targeted growth of selected inpatient services, and admission trends were changing. The demographics of its service area suggested overall growth would continue.

Applying Evidence-Based Management

Step 1: Formulating the Research Question

This project used evidence-based management techniques to respond to the problem of matching bed capacity to current and future needs. A steering committee specified the following research question: *Over the next three to five years,*

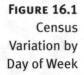

FIGURE 16.1
Census
Variation by
Day of Week

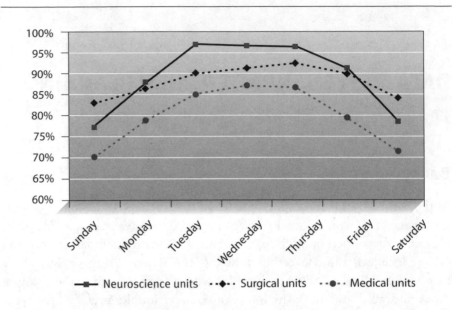

how many beds will Acme need, by service and level of care (general, intermediate, telemetry, and critical care), and what bed stack assignments will best accommodate current and future requirements with as little reassignment as possible?

The steering committee was led by the chief operating officer/executive vice president, the senior vice presidents of nursing and operations, the vice president of facilities, and representative division directors and medical directors, and aided by expert consultants.

Step 2: Acquiring Research Information

The steering committee projected future bed needs by evaluating current inpatient volume and bed utilization, reviewing strategic and business plans for the patient care services, leading user-group discussions to identify unit assets and deficiencies, and identifying anticipated changes in utilization and optimal unit attributes.

Inpatient Data

The consultants first collected discharge data—patient volume and patient days—from Acme's financial database for the prior 24-month period. Data were sorted by the discharging physician and assigned to the corresponding clinical service. Growth projections, estimated shifts in care locations, and market erosion would be applied to these data to predict future need. The team also collected bed utilization data, by service and by care level, which identified overall and service-specific utilization, and day-of-the-week variation (see Figure 16.1).

Facility and Functional Assessment

The consultants also convened user-group meetings to identify unit assets and deficiencies, both in the facility and in operational models. Discussions emphasized optimal unit attributes and adjacencies (which services needed to be located near which other services), healthcare trends that might affect admissions, and possible changes in utilization of critical care, telemetry, and progressive care beds. User groups consisted of physicians, nursing directors and managers, and product line managers.

Facility data regarding unit locations, configurations, and conditions also were collected. Unique unit features, such as the ratio of single- to double-occupancy rooms, telemetry capacity, number of isolation rooms, and so on, would be needed when unit reassignments were considered.

Benchmarks and Projections

If available, national standards or expected targets were compared with Acme Medical Center's admission patterns, bed utilization, and lengths of stay.

Unlike financial feasibility calculations, capacity planning can be based on various scenarios, representing limited, moderate, or aggressive growth. To best represent potential future conditions, these scenarios should integrate findings from several analyses:

- Projected usage by residents in the hospital's primary and secondary markets (expressed as hospital days or procedures per 1,000 population)
- Predicted or known changes in the market (e.g., closure of trauma centers or introduction of open-heart surgery)
- Anticipated changes in healthcare delivery (e.g., a shift from inpatient to outpatient settings or vice versa)
- Evaluation of historical growth
- Recent, approved, and anticipated physician recruitment, including anticipated discharge and procedure volumes for these physicians over time, whether the hospital capacity reflects these increases in demand, and whether business and marketing plans are in place to generate referrals to these new physicians

The Acme team took these factors into account and projected bed requirements by applying growth and erosion estimates developed by the hospital's planning staff to current inpatient data.

Step 3: Assessing the Validity, Quality, and Applicability of the Evidence

The user groups raised numerous important issues the consultants had to consider. Users believed Acme had:

- too few single-occupancy and isolation rooms, with many isolation rooms too small (approximately 100 square feet) for needed equipment and supplies;
- too few step-down beds, making discharge from critical care difficult;
- too few medicine beds, with overflow patients from the medical service distributed throughout the towers; medical staff reported having difficulty managing these dispersed patients, and surgery staff had trouble admitting patients to surgical units because beds were filled with medicine patients;
- too few critical care beds; staff had difficulty arranging admission to another service's ICU bed; beds were sometimes held for a potential patient while an actual patient waited in the emergency department;
- too few resources overall—beds, nurses, procedure space, and outpatient services—for the growing patient volume and to support the hospital's physician recruitment goals;
- "rules" for bed use that were inconsistent and changing; and
- increasing difficulty accepting transfers from other hospitals, due to capacity constraints.

To address these concerns, the consultants began an in-depth analysis of the hospital's data.

Discharge Data

During the 12 months prior to the study, Acme Medical Center discharged almost 34,000 patients, who accumulated more than 211,000 patient days and had an average length of stay (ALOS) of 6.2 days (Table 16.1).

The consultants quickly recognized that ALOS for adult services was significantly above the expected length of stay calculated from national benchmarks, which set expected lengths of stay of 5.58 days for all adult medical-surgical services. Although lengths of stay for surgical services and neuroscience unit services were approximately a half to a full day longer than the standard, the length of stay for medical services, 3.33 days longer than the standard, was the greatest deviation. Length- of-stay targets were developed for all services that exceeded the standards. Targets assumed that lengths of stay would be reduced by half of the variance between the actual and benchmark lengths of stay.

Inpatient Census Data

The consultants reviewed unit census data for the same 12-month period. (These data varied slightly from the discharge data.) They assessed not only average bed utilization, but also the average census by day of the week, to confirm a staff theory that census peaked Tuesdays through Thursdays. The team focused primarily on medical and surgical beds, assuming that

TABLE 16.1
Acme Medical
Center
Discharge Data

	Cases	ALOS	Patient Days
Medicine	6,985	9.85	70,266
Neurosciences	2,467	6.23	15,367
Surgery	10,831	5.57	60,300
Med-Surg Subtotal	*20,283*	*7.14*	*145,933*
Obstetrics	4,506	3.10	13,969
Pediatrics	7,679	4.81	36,901
Psychiatry	1,462	9.90	14,470
Total	*33,930*	*6.20*	*211,273*

ALOS: average length of stay

the psychiatric, obstetrical, and pediatric units were not used regularly as substitutes for the medical and surgical services or to accommodate overflow from these units.

Average utilization on the medical and surgical general care units was high, ranging from 76 to 94 percent, while average utilization for all medical and surgical units was 86 percent. Midweek utilization for medical-surgical units averaged 90 percent, declining on weekends to 81 percent.

The surgical units had more weekday variation than the medical units but lower utilization overall.

Adult Critical Care Utilization

Average utilization of the medical-surgical critical care beds was 86 percent, with individual units averaging from 83 to 91 percent. The midweek average was 90 percent, compared to a weekend average of 82 percent. Adult critical care days totaled 26,400—15.2 percent of total acute care days. The percentage utilization at Acme was below the 50th percentile for major teaching hospitals. (See Figure 16.2.)

National data indicate that critical care bed utilization has been relatively stable since the late 1990s (Solucient, LLC 2007). Large hospitals, hospitals in urban settings, and teaching hospitals deliver a higher percentage of critical care than the average hospital. In 2004, in hospitals with more than 400 beds, critical care accounted for a median of 17.4 percent of patient days, and in major teaching hospitals, it accounted for a median of 18.5 percent. In general, critical care utilization is 30 to 40 percent higher in hospitals where care is aggressively managed and lengths of stay are shorter. As length of stay is reduced, house-wide patient acuity is increased. Thus, efforts to reduce lengths of stay may increase the number of critical care beds needed.

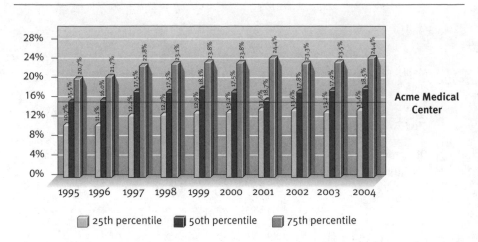

FIGURE 16.2
Percentage of
Patient Care
Days Delivered
in Critical Care
Among Major
U.S. Teaching
Hospitals

Bed Requirements for Current Patient Volume

Bed requirements were calculated using an 80 percent utilization target for
all units except psychiatry, which had a 90 percent utilization target. On the
basis of these targets, in the preceding year, adult medical and surgical services
were short 27 beds—essentially a full nursing unit (Table 16.2). Obstetrics
and psychiatry had minor deficiencies, and pediatrics had a surplus of beds.

The utilization targets used for inpatient bed planning typically range
between 80 and 85 percent. These targets take into account variables such
as gender placement, need for isolation beds, time required to ready beds
for new patients, and seasonal and day-of-the-week variations. At Acme
Medical Center, less than a third of the general care beds were in single
rooms, while the trend in inpatient facilities is toward 100 percent single-
occupancy rooms to accommodate the equipment and staff required to
care for sicker patients, the shifting of care to the bedside, the need to
reduce nosocomial infections, an increase in isolation requirements, and
patient expectations. A lower utilization rate target is needed when the
majority of beds are configured as doubles because the second bed in the
room is not always "usable," due to various factors.

Future Demand for Inpatient Beds

Planning efforts and capital investments should support strategic initiatives
and reflect strategic priorities. Strategic initiatives at Acme that the consultants recognized would directly or indirectly affect inpatient bed utilization included the following:

• A new chairman for neurosurgery had joined the staff in the fall and was
aggressively recruiting clinical staff, which would increase demand for
neuroscience ICU and step-down beds.

TABLE 16.2
Current Bed
Needs Versus
Actual
Allocation

	Beds Allocated	Average Daily Census	Bed Need at 80%	Variance
Surgical units	168	134.2	168	0
Medical units	188	164.0	205	−17
Neuroscience unit	32	28.6	35.8	−4
Adult General Care Subtotal	*388*	*327*	*409*	*−21*
Critical care	84	72.3	90	−6
Med-Surg Total	*472*	*399*	*499*	*−27*
Obstetrics	46	38.3	47.8	−2
Pediatrics				
• NICU	48	34.0	42.5	6
• General care	76	56.4	70.5	5
• Pediatric ICU	14	10.7	13.4	1
Pediatric Subtotal	*138*	*101*	*126*	*12*
Psychiatry (bed need at 90%)	42	39.6	44	−2
Total	*698*	*578*		

- Interventional radiology was experiencing an increase in patient volume. Although many of the cases were outpatients, interventional radiology involves complex procedures that need short-stay or 23-hour post-procedure care with a high level of nursing.
- The oncology unit was frequently full, and patients were boarded on other units. The ALOS for oncology exceeded the expected by more than a day. The service staff reported difficulty in managing patients dispersed throughout the bed towers.
- Pediatrics was recruiting a new chair, who would likely attempt to expand this service.
- The city had requested that all hospitals decrease the number of times they place their emergency service on ambulance diversion. At Acme, diversion typically occurred because ICU beds were full.

In addition, several clinical services were expected to experience a shift in patient volume:

- Urology and gynecology were moving to outpatient and short-stay procedures, which would increase the need for 23-hour beds.
- The introduction of proton-beam radiation therapy at a competing hospital could decrease the volume of prostate cancer patients treated at Acme.

TABLE 16.3
Five-Year
Volume
Projections

	Year 1 Projections			Year 2 Projections			Year 3 Projections			Year 4 Projections			Year 5 Projections		
	Pt. Volume	Pt. Days	ALOS	Pt. Volume	Pt. Days	ALOS	Pt. Volume	Pt. Days	ALOS	Pt. Volume	Pt. Days	ALOS	Pt. Volume	Pt. Days	ALOS
Surgical															
Cardiothoracic	1,793	14,874	8.29	1,779	14,726	8.28	1,765	14,608	8.28	1,765	14,608	8.28	1,765	14,608	8.28
Gastrointestinal	2,554	10,532	4.12	2,687	10,679	3.97	2,826	11,043	3.91	3,030	11,484	3.79	3,212	12,173	3.79
General surgery	2,746	16,579	6.04	2,798	16,744	5.98	2,851	16,945	5.94	2,905	17,216	5.93	2,960	17,544	5.93
GYN	2,832	8,475	2.99	2,832	8,255	2.91	2,832	8,023	2.83	2,832	7,943	2.80	2,832	7,943	2.80
Transplant	1,205	9,510	7.89	1,304	11,174	8.57	1,437	12,739	8.87	1,523	13,274	8.72	1,584	13,805	8.72
Subtotal	*11,130*	*59,970*	*5.39*	*11,400*	*61,578*	*5.40*	*11,711*	*63,358*	*5.41*	*12,055*	*64,525*	*5.35*	*12,353*	*66,073*	*5.35*
Medical															
General	2,374	17,090	7.20	2,469	16,748	6.78	2,563	16,413	6.40	2,661	16,085	6.05	2,746	16,600	6.05
Cardiology	1,928	10,194	5.29	2,038	10,011	4.91	2,124	9,830	4.63	2,213	9,653	4.36	2,297	10,020	4.36
HIV	1,012	10,126	10.01	1,022	10,014	9.80	1,032	9,834	9.53	1,043	9,657	9.26	1,053	9,754	9.26
Infectious disease	1,408	8,897	6.32	1,425	8,799	6.17	1,440	8,702	6.05	1,454	8,607	5.92	1,454	8,607	5.92
Oncology	1,414	10,250	7.25	1,460	10,066	6.90	1,501	9,884	6.59	1,543	9,707	6.29	1,586	9,978	6.29
Pulmonary	1,573	12,367	7.86	1,595	12,367	7.75	1,636	12,243	7.48	1,679	12,121	7.22	1,713	12,363	7.22
Subtotal	*9,709*	*68,924*	*7.10*	*10,009*	*68,005*	*6.79*	*10,296*	*66,906*	*6.50*	*10,593*	*65,830*	*6.22*	*10,849*	*67,322*	*6.21*
Neurosciences															
Neurology	1,643	7,757	4.72	1,857	7,835	4.22	1,935	7,913	4.09	1,993	8,071	4.05	2,049	8,297	4.05
Neurosurgery	1,064	7,598	7.14	1,075	7,545	7.02	1,096	7,545	6.88	1,107	7,545	6.82	1,118	7,621	6.82
Subtotal	*2,707*	*15,355*	*5.67*	*2,932*	*15,380*	*5.25*	*3,031*	*15,458*	*5.10*	*3,100*	*15,616*	*5.04*	*3,167*	*15,918*	*5.03*
Med-Surg Total	*23,546*	*144,249*	*6.13*	*24,341*	*144,963*	*5.96*	*25,038*	*145,722*	*5.82*	*25,748*	*145,971*	*5.67*	*26,369*	*149,313*	*5.66*

TABLE 16.4
Five-Year
Projected Bed
Needs, Based
on Length of
Stay Targets

	Current Beds	Year 1	Year 3	Year 5	Variance at Year 5
Surgery	204	205	217	226	22
Medicine	220	236	229	231	11
Neuroscience	48	53	53	55	7
Adult Med-Surg Subtotal	*472*	*494*	*499*	*512*	*40*
Obstetrics	46	48	48	48	2
NICU	48	42	42	42	–6
Pediatrics	90	84	84	86	–4
Psychiatry	42	44	44	50	8

TABLE 16.5
Five-Year
Projected Bed
Need with
Acme's Existing
Lengths-of-Stay

	Current Beds	Year 1	Year 3	Year 5	Variance at Year 5
Surgery	204	212	224	236	32
Medicine	220	245	260	273	53
Neuroscience	48	57	63	66	18
Adult Med-Surg Subtotal	*472*	*514*	*547*	*575*	*103*
Obstetrics	46	48	48	48	2
NICU	48	42	42	42	–6
Pediatrics	90	87	92	94	4
Psychiatry	42	44	44	44	2

To aid the project, the hospital's planning staff made five-year projections of patient volume. These projections incorporated estimated growth and erosion in patient volume and were tested against market-growth and market-share assumptions (Table 16.3). Volume projections were based on the assumption that bed capacity would not limit growth. The *theoretical* five-year bed capacity needs, based on national length-of-stay norms, are shown in Table 16.4.

Challenges and Opportunities

Length-of-Stay Reductions

Prior efforts to reduce lengths of stay at Acme had been only marginally successful. If these metrics remained stable, the theoretical projections would be insufficient, and future beds would need to increase significantly (Table 16.5). At the end of five years, instead of being 40 beds short, Acme's medical-surgical units would be more than 100 beds short.

Bed Gridlock

Frequently, Acme's nurses struggled to vacate a bed to accommodate patient placement needs. They had to move a current patient, a process often impeded by the movement of another patient, which was again impeded by yet another patient move, resulting in "bed gridlock." Excessive resources were being expended in these moves (which also are associated with a high risk of various kinds of clinical errors), and the consultants believed the encumbered patient flow was probably extending the ALOS, further increasing bed demand. Gridlock at Acme resulted from:

- high bed utilization, particularly in critical care;
- too few single rooms;
- too few beds with monitoring capacity; and
- other operational issues, such as unbalanced procedure schedules, holding beds, and inaccurate or untimely communication.

Census Peaks

The consultants observed that balancing admissions more evenly across the seven days of the week, or at least from Monday through Friday, would ease bed demand. They concluded that the surgical, radiology, and cardiology procedure schedules should be reviewed in an attempt to distribute inpatient cases more evenly and, if possible, to distribute them according to their anticipated lengths of stay to more evenly distribute the inpatient patient-day volume.

23-Hour Unit

Outpatients requiring short-term, highly technical, or complex nursing care were either admitted to an inpatient bed or cared for in the emergency department or post-anesthesia care unit. Providing an alternative site for this care could decrease the demand for inpatient beds. The consultants concluded that a 23-hour care unit would meet the needs of these patients and would not have to be located in one of the bed towers. Space adjacent to one of the procedure areas or easily accessible from an entrance would be suitable.

Step 4: Presenting the Evidence

At this point the consultants presented their findings to the steering committee for review, discussion, and revision. The committee made only minor changes. The findings were then presented to the medical department and service line chiefs and the nursing directors. Following these meetings, presentations were given to the nurse managers, and an open meeting was held for physicians. Buy-in from these groups had to be secured before the findings were applied to the development of bed stack options. If staff disagreed with the data analysis and conclusions, solutions developed from them would not be accepted as valid.

Although the meetings produced significant discussion and questions about the data and the methodology, only one significant revision was required. The discharge data were originally sorted into service cohorts by diagnosis-related group assignments, but the physicians requested that they be developed on the basis of the specialty of the discharging physician. The concept of "discharging physician of record" was used for other purposes in both the medical center and medical school, and physicians were comfortable with how that variable was determined. Meeting participants acknowledged that both methods of assigning patients had flaws, and neither was superior to the other, so discharge data were re-sorted as requested.

Step 5: Using the Findings to Develop and Select a Solution

Planning Guidelines and Priorities

Early in the process, the steering committee drafted planning guidelines and priorities to frame how the consultants would approach the challenges. These guidelines indicated that bed stack options should strive to address these principles:

1. Align bed assignment/unit cohorts with current and projected bed requirements:

   - Provide sufficient beds to accommodate the growth anticipated for surgery and neurosciences.
   - Define specific unit locations for services emphasized in the strategy agenda, such as transplantation and neurosciences.
   - Identify unit locations for services that admit the majority of patients in each department.

2. Maintain or create departmental horizontal adjacencies between inpatient, outpatient, and administrative spaces, where possible. For example, cardiac surgery and neurosciences had horizontal adjacencies. (Because neurosciences needed additional beds, and no growth was possible on its floor, relocation of general care neurosciences beds was likely.)

3. Provide adequate critical care beds to match anticipated growth in patient volume.

4. Establish a reasonable implementation sequence:
   - Implementation should result in as little disruption to the workforce and patients as possible.

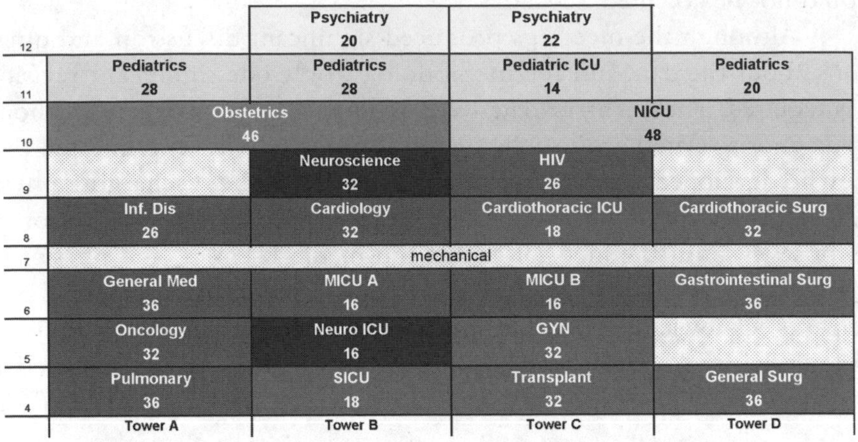

FIGURE 16.3
Configuration of Bed Stack at the Start of the Redesign Project

- The number of unit relocations should be minimized.
- Units required to relocate should have to do so only once in the next five years.
- The reuse of the inpatient facility in its current configuration should be maximized.

Planning Guidelines: Alternative Example

Planning guidelines are unique and specific to each hospital. A similar hospital drafted the following guidelines, which are quite different, yet equally appropriate.

- The right bed should be available at the right time.
- Beds are an organization-wide resource.
- Changing practice patterns and rising patient expectations increase the need for more single-occupancy rooms. The higher incidence of drug-resistant infections also is escalating the need for single and isolation rooms.
- Staff levels (physician and nursing) must be kept in equilibrium with patient volumes and care-level requirements.
- Inpatient space should be flexible, multiuse, and adaptable for the many changes anticipated in care delivery and patient volumes.
- Investment on the main campus should comply with "highest and best reuse" of the buildings.

Current Configuration

Figure 16.3 and Table 16.6 show the unit locations and bed allocation as they existed at the start of the project.

	Beds Allocated		
Service	General Care	Critical Care	Total
Surgery	168	36	204
Medicine	188	32	220
Neuroscience	32	16	48
Adult Med-Surg Subtotal	*388*	*84*	*472*
Obstetrics	46	0	46
NICU	0	48	48
Pediatrics	76	14	90
Psychiatry	42	0	42

TABLE 16.6
Bed Allocation by Unit at the Start of the Redesign Project

In addition to the guidelines and priorities cited above, the steering committee had the following objectives as it began to develop bed stack options:

• Increase step-down bed capacity.
• Increase critical care bed capacity, specifically in relationship to overall bed increases.
• Increase single-occupancy and isolation rooms.

Constraints in developing the bed stack options were: (a) because beds are so heavily utilized, a unit could not be closed for renovation or reconfiguration until additional beds were added, and (b) towers A and D were not well suited for critical care units. Making planning somewhat easier, floors 5 and 9 in Tower D were decommissioned inpatient units that could be used after only moderate reconfiguration. Unit 9A also was a decommissioned inpatient unit, but significant reconfiguration of this unit had occurred, and it would have been expensive to reclaim it for inpatient functions.

Several short-term (three-year horizon) and long-term (five years and beyond) options were developed and evaluated. Solutions selected for implementation are described below.

Short-Term Solution

The steering committee ultimately recommended that:

1. Floors 5 and 9 in Tower D be vacated and renovated for return to inpatient care;
2. The neuroscience general care beds be relocated to 4A, adjacent to the neurology ICU;

FIGURE 16.4
Revised Bed
Stack: Short-Term
Reconfiguration

	Tower A	Tower B	Tower C	Tower D
12		Psychiatry 20	Psychiatry 22	
11	Pediatrics 28	Pediatrics 28	Pediatric ICU 14	Pediatrics 20
10	Obstetrics 46		NICU 48	
9		Pulmonary 36	HIV 26	Oncology 32
8	Inf. Dis 26	General Medicine 32	Cardiothoracic ICU 18	Cardiothoracic Surg 32
7	mechanical			
6	Cardiology 36	MICU A 16	MICU B 16	Medical Step-down 26
5	Neuroscience 32	Neuro ICU 16	GYN 32	Gastrointestinal Surg 36
4	Surgical Step-down 26	SICU 18	Transplant 32	General Surg 36

3. Two step-down units, each with 26 single-occupancy beds, be created on 4A and 6D, immediately adjacent to the surgical ICU and the medical ICU-B; and

4. Cardiology be relocated to 6A, since a high percentage of these patients end up being cared for in the medical ICU.

The impact of these recommendations is shown in Figure 16.4 and Tables 16.7 and 16.8. If ALOS targets were achieved, the proposed short-term bed stack would exceed the Year 3 requirements for the adult medical and surgical services (Table 16.7). If *no* decrease in ALOS occurred, the additional 58 beds would be insufficient to meet the Year 3 demand (Table 16.8).

ICU Beds

The addition of 58 adult medical and surgical beds without a corresponding increase in critical care beds decreased the ratio of ICU beds from 15.2 to 13.7 per 100 medical-surgical beds. The planners hoped that, for the short term, the addition of 52 step-down beds would compensate.

Longer-Term Solution

The steering committee also recommended a longer-term solution, taking into account the short-term steps already accomplished:

1. Construct four new floors in towers B and C, to include two floors of inpatient beds, one shelled floor, and one floor to house mechanical equipment.

2. Configure the new units on 14B and C and 15B and C with 24 single-occupancy rooms each.

3. Reconfigure double-occupancy rooms on the remaining units for single occupancy.

TABLE 16.7
Year 3 Beds
Proposed and
Required, if
ALOS Targets
Were Achieved

	Beds Needed If ALOS Targets Were Achieved	Beds Proposed under Short-Term Reconfiguration	Variance
Surgery	217	230	13
Medicine	229	246	17
Neuroscience	53	48	−5
Adult Med-Surg Subtotal	499	524	25
Obstetrics	48	46	−2
NICU	42	48	6
Pediatrics	84	90	6
Psychiatry	44	42	−2

TABLE 16.8
Year 3 Beds
Proposed and
Required with
No Change in
ALOS

	Beds Needed If ALOS Targets Were NOT Achieved	Beds Proposed under Short-Term Reconfiguration	Variance
Surgery	224	230	6
Medicine	260	246	−14
Neuroscience	63	48	−15
Adult Med-Surg Subtotal	547	524	−23
Obstetrics	48	46	−2
NICU	42	48	6
Pediatrics	92	90	−2
Psychiatry	44	42	−2

4. Assign an additional neurosciences unit on 5C, increasing its bed allocation and introducing step-down beds.
5. Create a third 18-bed medical ICU on 9C.
6. Create a new cardiothoracic ICU on 9C, and relocate cardiothoracic general care beds to 9D.
7. Create a second surgical ICU on 6B.
8. Upgrade to selected units following the completion of new construction.

Again, the impact on bed stack (Figure 16.5) and bed capacity is shown both with and without meeting ALOS targets. If length-of-stay targets were achieved, the proposed bed stack would exceed the Year 5 requirements for adult medical and surgical services (Table 16.9). And two shelled

FIGURE 16.5
Revised Bed
Stack: Longer-
Term Solution

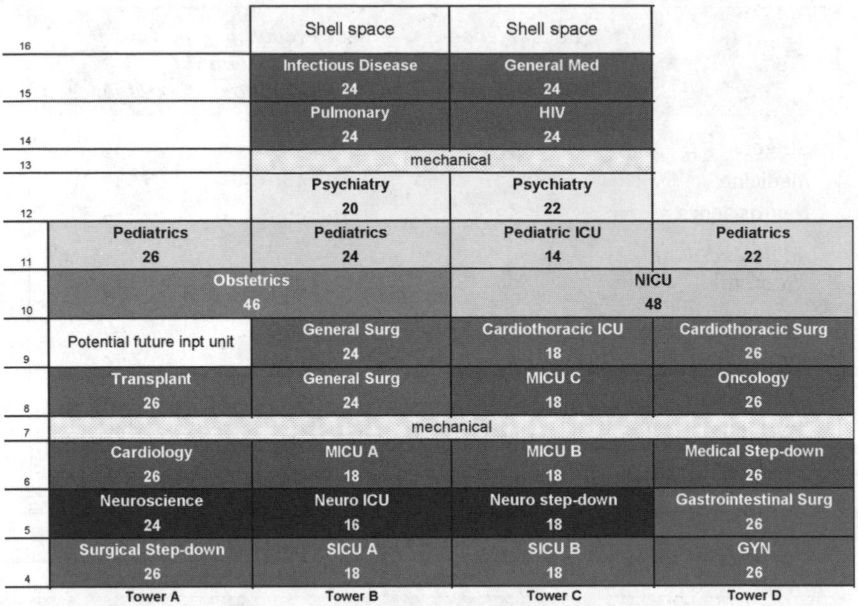

	Shell space	Shell space	
16			
15	Infectious Disease 24	General Med 24	
14	Pulmonary 24	HIV 24	
13	mechanical		
12	Psychiatry 20	Psychiatry 22	
11	Pediatrics 26	Pediatrics 24	Pediatric ICU 14	Pediatrics 22
10	Obstetrics 46		NICU 48	
9	Potential future inpt unit	General Surg 24	Cardiothoracic ICU 18	Cardiothoracic Surg 26
8	Transplant 26	General Surg 24	MICU C 18	Oncology 26
7	mechanical			
6	Cardiology 26	MICU A 18	MICU B 18	Medical Step-down 26
5	Neuroscience 24	Neuro ICU 16	Neuro step-down 18	Gastrointestinal Surg 26
4	Surgical Step-down 26	SICU A 18	SICU B 18	GYN 26
	Tower A	Tower B	Tower C	Tower D

FIGURE 16.6
Alternative
Long-Term Bed
Stack

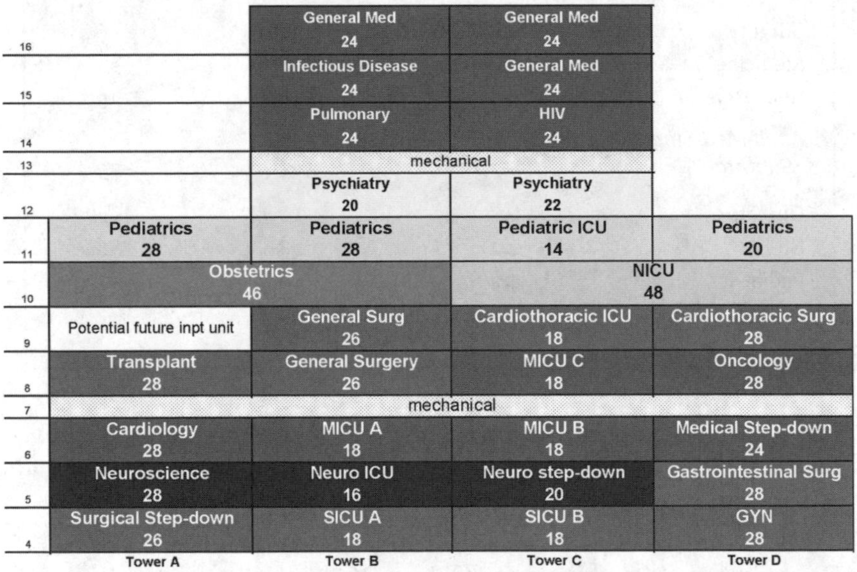

	General Med 24	General Med 24	
16	Infectious Disease 24	General Med 24	
15	Pulmonary 24	HIV 24	
14			
13	mechanical		
12	Psychiatry 20	Psychiatry 22	
11	Pediatrics 28	Pediatrics 28	Pediatric ICU 14	Pediatrics 20
10	Obstetrics 46		NICU 48	
9	Potential future inpt unit	General Surg 26	Cardiothoracic ICU 18	Cardiothoracic Surg 28
8	Transplant 28	General Surgery 26	MICU C 18	Oncology 28
7	mechanical			
6	Cardiology 28	MICU A 18	MICU B 18	Medical Step-down 24
5	Neuroscience 28	Neuro ICU 16	Neuro step-down 20	Gastrointestinal Surg 28
4	Surgical Step-down 26	SICU A 18	SICU B 18	GYN 28
	Tower A	Tower B	Tower C	Tower D

units, able to accommodate 48 additional beds, and unit 9A would be available for future growth. But if Acme were unsuccessful in reaching the ALOS targets, the proposed long-term strategy would fail to meet projected bed needs (Table 16.10).

The longer-term strategy also achieved an increase in critical care capacity, to accompany the increase in general care beds. The ratio of adult

	Beds Needed If ALOS Targets Are Achieved	Beds Proposed Under Longer-Term Reconfiguration	Variance
Surgery	226	232	6
Medicine	231	228	−3
Neuroscience	55	58	3
Adult Med-Surg Subtotal	512	518	6
Obstetrics	48	46	−2
NICU	42	48	6
Pediatrics	86	86	0
Psychiatry	50	42	−8

TABLE 16.9
Year 5 Beds Proposed and Required, if ALOS Targets Were Achieved

	Beds Needed If ALOS Targets Are NOT Achieved	Beds Proposed Under Longer-Term Reconfiguration	Variance
Surgery	236	232	−4
Medicine	273	228	−45
Neuroscience	66	58	−8
Adult Med-Surg Subtotal	575	518	−57
Obstetrics	48	46	−2
NICU	42	48	6
Pediatrics	94	86	−8
Psychiatry	44	42	−2

TABLE 16.10
Year 5 Beds Proposed and Required with No Change in ALOS

acute care to critical care beds would be increased from 15.2 to 20.5 per hundred beds—slightly above the median for academic medical centers. Step-down beds would not increase from the number proposed for the short term. If additional step-down capacity were required, 4D would be the next surgical step-down unit, and 6A or 8D would be the next medical step-down unit. Both would be adjacent to corresponding critical care units.

Alternative Longer-Term Bed Stack Arrangement

In this alternative bed stack arrangement, which achieves an even larger number of new beds, Acme has the option of either completing the shelled units or maintaining a subset of beds in double-occupancy rooms. A mix

TABLE 16.11
Alternative
Configuration
of Year 5 Beds,
No Change in
ALOS

	Beds Needed If ALOS Targets Are NOT Achieved	Number of Beds under Alternative Longer-Term Configuration	Variance
Surgery	236	244	8
Medicine	273	278	5
Neuroscience	66	64	−2
Adult Med-Surg Subtotal	*575*	*586*	*11*
Obstetrics	48	46	−2
NICU	42	48	6
Pediatrics	94	90	−4
Psychiatry	44	42	−2

of these two approaches is presented in Figure 16.6. In this configuration, the two shelled units on 16 are put in use, and double-occupancy rooms are maintained on most general care units. This set of changes results in a slight excess of beds in nearly all units, even if ALOS targets are not reached (Table 16.11).

Conclusion

Medical centers are in a constant state of change—new programs, new physicians, new technologies, new treatments, and new kinds of patients. A thorough understanding of the rationale and principles in assigning units, as demonstrated in the above evidence-based process, leads to more intelligent accommodation of both expected growth and unanticipated patient volume, unlike the common practice of "squeezing it in somewhere" and repenting at leisure.

Reference

Solucient, LLC. 2007. *The Comparative Performance of U.S. Hospitals: The Sourcebook. 2001–2006.* New York: Solucient, LLC.

USING EVIDENCE-BASED MANAGEMENT TO IMPROVE OPERATING ROOM SCHEDULING

Megin Wolfman

Background

Operating room (OR) time is an inherently limited resource for which demand is high. Hospital administrators face considerable pressure to allocate OR time efficiently and streamline the scheduling process, and many have adopted block scheduling to respond to this pressure. Block scheduling, when executed effectively, can improve overall OR efficiency by (a) allocating time according to historical utilization patterns and expectations of future needs and (b) allowing day-to-day schedule variations to be managed locally.

> **What Is Block Scheduling?**
>
> With block scheduling, a block of OR time—either specific rooms or set hours—is allocated to a surgical service, group of surgeons, or individual surgeons.

Block scheduling can yield several advantages over individual, or "open access," scheduling, in which surgeons do their own scheduling. Open access scheduling works best in hospitals that have lower surgical volume and relatively predictable case types; in tertiary care medical centers, however, it soon becomes unwieldy and may require significant human resource, technology, and other infrastructure investments. Challenges of open access scheduling include the following:

- The system for "real-time" scheduling can be expensive to develop and maintain.
- Accountability for productivity and workflow is too decentralized.
- If surgeons don't complete all the required scheduling paperwork, last-minute cancellations can occur, which are disruptive to patients, their surgeons, and the OR staff.
- Its unpredictability makes managing the schedules of OR staff and the availability of other resources difficult.

- Add-on and emergency cases can be difficult to accommodate.
- Less desirable time slots are underused.
- Surgeons prefer schedules that are consistent over time and allow them to perform multiple procedures back to back.

Environmental Considerations

Although block scheduling has become a relatively common practice among the nation's leading hospitals, it does not directly address significant environmental pressures on OR efficiency that concern OR managers. These pressures are discussed below:

Capacity and Strategic Growth

The number of surgical procedures may increase, but at any point in time, a hospital's OR capacity is fixed. Managers are challenged to accommodate not only greater overall volume, but also the "right" volume (e.g., strategically or financially desirable surgical services).

Organizational Challenges and Political Considerations

A block schedule is not immutable. It will need to be revised periodically, which requires that changes be implemented appropriately and with the concordance of hospital leadership. Not only must the manager overcome organizational inertia to change, but he or she also may face pushback from departments or surgical groups that feel they are "losers" in the reallocation of time. For example, if a hospital department has recruited new surgeons with the promise of a certain amount of OR time, it can see the reallocation as jeopardizing its strategic growth priorities.

Logistical Challenges

Logistical challenges, such as accommodation of add-on and emergency cases outside of normally allocated blocks, pose a continual challenge to efficient OR use. Consistency over time is what allows advance scheduling, which increases satisfaction of surgeons and patients and improves efficiency.

Regulatory and Patient Care Considerations

Not all ORs are equal: Short-term facility and equipment constraints may limit the flexibility of a particular OR. Uncertainty about the future demand for certain types of procedures further complicates efforts to predict schedules longer term.

The Case: Block Scheduling at Memorial Hospital

Memorial Hospital operates 19 inpatient ORs, 15 ambulatory ORs, and a variety of other procedure suites. The ORs have relied on a block scheduling model dating back more than a decade. Through 2005, the original block schedule remained relatively unchanged, with no department gaining, losing, or even shifting its allocated time in any meaningful way. There were no unallocated time blocks, performance review processes, or methods to accommodate surgical recruits brought into the hospital as a result of various departments' strategic commitments. During 2005, several forces converged to threaten this system:

- The ORs were stretched to capacity, relative to their average monthly volume (then in excess of 2,000 cases), current levels of efficiency, and formal hours of operation (eight-hour blocks, Monday through Friday).
- Almost all lower-acuity procedures had been moved to other sites, and the types of procedures still performed in the main ORs needed to stay there.
- Since all of the hours were blocked, the ORs could not accommodate a growing number of emergency and add-on cases, nor could they continue to absorb the steady year-to-year increase in volume (nearly 10 percent) and the demands of newly recruited surgeons.

These conditions required longer-than-optimal hours of operation and threatened to limit additional growth, which, although not quantified, was expected to remain consistent with the hospital's recent trends. The hospital would need several years to solve the problem by building new, expanded surgical facilities. OR managers and clinical leadership began discussing ways to improve the scheduling system and agreed on the need to reallocate the current OR blocks—not merely as a onetime fix, but as an ongoing process to optimize OR scheduling. To make this reallocation successful, they took an evidence-based, objective, data-driven approach that was fair to all stakeholders.

Applying Evidence-Based Management

Step 1: Formulating the Research Question

OR managers believed they first needed to understand the current level of efficiency in the OR schedule before they could identify and implement improvements. Their guiding research questions became: What is the current level of block utilization, what is the variation across departments, and what are the opportunities for improving overall utilization and minimizing interdepartmental variation?

FIGURE 17.1
OR Productivity
Indicators

FIGURE 17.1
OR Productivity
Indicators

Step 2: Acquiring the Evidence

Managers conducted several concurrent analyses to gather evidence related to their questions.

Literature and Industry-Based Best Practices

Managers researched scheduling structures at peer hospitals across the country through extensive literature searches, discussions with several national associations, and informal networking.[1] While this research confirmed that block OR scheduling was relatively commonplace—particularly at academic medical centers—managers found few formal evaluations, benchmarking projects, or recommendations regarding block allocation and reallocation. The problem of OR productivity was widely discussed, but systemic or evidence-based solutions were not.

Evaluation of Current OR Efficiency—Balanced Scorecard

OR managers also set about examining their own data. They developed a balanced scorecard for the ORs, focusing on productivity indicators (Figure 17.1). This effort yielded robust trend data on many efficiency measures related to block utilization, such as room utilization, OR turnaround times, percentage of first cases that started on time, and recovery room availability. These metrics helped in diagnosing root causes of efficiency and evaluating overall OR productivity.

FIGURE 17.2
Quarterly
Departmental
Reports

MEMORIAL HOSPITAL
OR BLOCK UTILIZATION SUMMARY BY <u>DEPARTMENT</u>
Q4 2005

DEPT OF SURGERY

I. CURRENT BLOCK ALLOCATIONS

		HRS/WEEK				
		MON	TUE	WED	THU	FRI
	Inpatient	xx	xx	xx	xx	xx
	Ambulatory	xx	xx	xx	xx	xx

II. BLOCK UTILIZATION

		MONTHLY AVERAGE			Q4 2005	QTR AVERAGE BY DAY				
		OCT 05	NOV 05	DEC 05	AVE	MON	TUE	WED	THU	FRI
	Inpatient	xx%	xx%	xx%	xx%	xx%	xx%	xx%	xx%	xx%
	Ambulatory	xx%	xx%	xx%	xx%	xx%	xx%	xx%	xx%	xx%

III. CASE COUNT IN BLOCK

		MONTHLY AVE CASES			Q4 2005	QTR AVERAGE BY DAY				
		OCT 05	NOV 05	DEC 05	AVE	MON	TUE	WED	THU	FRI
	Inpatient	xx	xx	xx	xx	xx	xx	xx	xx	xx
	Ambulatory	xx	xx	xx	xx	xx	xx	xx	xx	xx

IV. OUT-OF-BLOCK MINUTES

		MONTHLY TOTALS			Q4 2005	%	QTR AVERAGE BY DAY					
		OCT 05	NOV 05	DEC 05	AVE	SCHED	MON	TUE	WED	THU	FRI	SAT
IP	M-F BLOCK END-5:30	xx	xx	xx	xx		xx	xx	xx	xx	xx	xx
	M-F 5:30-10:00PM	xx	xx	xx	xx		xx	xx	xx	xx	xx	xx
	M-F 10:00PM-7:30AM	xx	xx	xx	xx		xx	xx	xx	xx	xx	xx
	SA-SU	xx	xx	xx	xx		xx	xx	xx	xx	xx	xx
	M-F PEAK OOB	xx	xx	xx	xx		xx	xx	xx	xx	xx	xx
	TOTAL	xx	xx	xx	xx		xx	xx	xx	xx	xx	xx
AMB	M-F BLOCK END-5:30	xx	xx	xx	xx		xx	xx	xx	xx	xx	xx
	M-F 5:30-10:00PM	xx	xx	xx	xx		xx	xx	xx	xx	xx	xx
	M-F 10:00PM-7:30AM	xx	xx	xx	xx		xx	xx	xx	xx	xx	xx
	SA-SU	xx	xx	xx	xx		xx	xx	xx	xx	xx	xx
	M-F PEAK OOB	xx	xx	xx	xx		xx	xx	xx	xx	xx	xx
	TOTAL	xx	xx	xx	xx		xx	xx	xx	xx	xx	xx

Notes:
> Block assumptions include adjustment for turnaround
> Case = patient in to patient out; data includes scheduled and unscheduled cases
> Utilization over 100% is possible only if a service is using rooms in addition to those formally allocated

Internal Database of Block Utilization

Managers built a data set that accurately illustrated the utilization of block time currently allocated to clinical departments. Summaries of these data provided managers and clinical leadership with much meaningful information, including variations in usage by day and time segment. Quarterly reports were developed for each department (Figure 17.2). Managers also developed an extensive catalog of data on individual surgeons, including intra-operative time in the departmental block. To enable direct, department-to-department comparisons, data were adjusted, according to industry standards, to account for variation in turnaround time and other factors outside the departments' control. Managers minimized the risk that data could be manipulated by hardwiring relevant entries (such as "time physician enters room") into the case protocols followed by OR staff.

Finally, managers analyzed each department's use of OR time *outside* its allocated block. In some cases, managers could simply accommodate a department's extra volume by formally extending its hours. But some departments with high out-of-block utilization had *low* block utilization, and, again, managers could make immediate improvements while continuing to evaluate longer-term reallocation issues. As shown in Figure 17.2, this out-of-block time was broken into meaningful subsets, including hours immediately following official operating time, and evening, overnight, and weekend hours. An additional category, "peak out-of-block" time, identified OR use during peak hours, when a department had no officially allocated block time.

Results Analysis

The initial in-block and out-of-block utilization analysis revealed various patterns:

- *Wide utilization variation across departments.* Several departments maintained reliably low utilization, while others continued to function above optimal levels.
- *Utilization variation across days, both within and between departments.* While demand was typically lowest on Fridays, other slumps appeared throughout the week.
- *Complementarity.* Periods of high utilization in one department often corresponded to periods of low utilization in another department.
- *Disproportionate out-of-block utilization.* Certain departments consistently underused their own time blocks but were high out-of-block users.
- *High in-block and out-of-block utilization.* Other departments maintained both high in-block and high out-of-block utilization consistently through the end of the evening out-of-block category.
- *Use of weekend hours.* One department had begun to use more Saturday hours while simultaneously optimizing its in-block utilization.

Research-Related Costs

Since internal staff conducted all the research and existing resources developed the OR dashboard, Memorial Hospital incurred minimal direct expense for data collection and evaluation. The only measurable incremental cost to the hospital was the expense (undetermined) associated with developing the block utilization database.

Steps 3 and 4: Assessing the Validity, Quality, and Applicability of the Evidence and Presenting the Evidence

Memorial Hospital relied on a long-standing and effective OR committee—consisting of the surgical chiefs of service, clinical OR management, and administrative leadership, including the chief medical officer, chief operating officer, and vice president of perioperative services—to guide policy. But because this group could not give sufficient attention to issues around scheduling and efficiency optimization, an OR executive committee[2] was created to address these and other key issues in greater depth.

To prevent bias in data interpretation, the OR executive committee first discussed and reached consensus on the way the research data were collected. It then viewed the preliminary departmental block utilization data and tested committee members' assumptions against those results. Data tracked separately by individual departments also were used to validate the new, broader data set. Finally, the committee assessed the data and the report formats to make sure they would clearly communicate the ration-

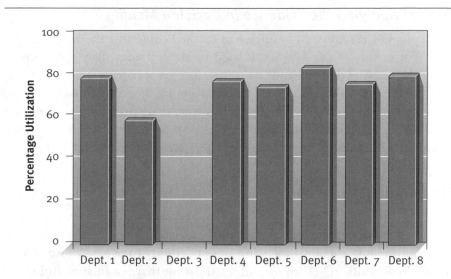

FIGURE 17.3
OR Block
Utilization,
Q3 2005

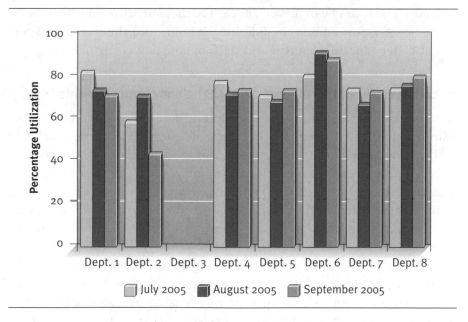

FIGURE 17.4
OR Block
Utilization by
month, Q3
2005

ale for future reallocation decisions to the OR committee as a whole, to individual surgeons, and to hospital leadership.

Figures 17.3 and 17.4 show the high-level summaries presented to the OR executive committee. The external research had uncovered no universal benchmarks of appropriate OR utilization because optimal levels depend on too many hospital-specific factors (Patterson 2004); therefore, the committee chose target ranges according to managers' expectations of "reasonable" utilization—75 to 85 percent for the inpatient suite and 70 to 80 percent for the ambulatory suite.

Step 5: Applying the Evidence in Decision Making

Once the OR executive committee had reached consensus about the quality and applicability of the data set, it tried to identify immediate solutions to meet the growing demand and to institute an appropriate, effective, and balanced policy for reallocating block OR time among departments based on the data set, which would resolve short-term inefficiencies from misallocation and provide the foundation for a long-term evaluation and reallocation process. To accomplish these tasks, it took two short-term actions, described below.

OR Schedule Extensions

The OR executive committee found that several departments were maximizing their block time, but also regularly extending beyond the 3:30 p.m. scheduled cutoff, thereby indicating an opportunity to extend those blocks, normally 8 hours, to 12 hours. After validating that seasonality and other factors were not significantly influencing usage and that future volumes were expected to remain strong, the OR executive committee formally extended one room by four hours in each of these departments. As a result, these departments could schedule longer hours and their OR managers could better allocate resources and staff, minimizing costly overtime.

Encouragement of Intradepartmental Efficiency Improvements

The OR executive committee also determined that opportunities for improvement existed in many departments—especially those that were underusing their block time and overusing out-of-block time. The OR executive committee recommended: (a) improved alignment of surgeon and departmental schedules; (b) advance department release of block time when appropriate (with departmental "credit" awarded if blocks were relinquished more than two weeks in advance); and (c) intradepartmental reallocations.

To support these actions, managers gave department chairs the OR dashboard, departmental block utilization summary reports, and surgeon-level utilization reports. Managers and analysts collaborated with departments as needed to interpret them and implement changes based on the data.

The OR executive committee then began developing a formal block reallocation policy, with these objectives:

- An objective, fair, and data-driven rationale for reallocations among departments;
- Experience-based utilization targets and thresholds;
- Flexibility to accommodate day-to-day schedule changes needed to accommodate emergency and add-on cases;
- Flexibility to accommodate hospital-wide strategic growth priorities; and
- Regular assessment and reallocation, as necessary.

Step 6: Evaluating Results and Making Improvements
Reallocations Implemented

The ongoing evaluation process resulted in reallocation involving four departments in January 2006, two of which lost four hours (half a block) per week, and two of which gained four hours per week. The director of perioperative services, representing the OR executive committee, met directly with the department chairs involved to review the policy and its implications in detail, reinforcing the non-punitive nature of the reallocation, as well as the potential for a department to regain its time in subsequent review cycles if its efficiency could be improved. OR managers then continued to track the efficiency metrics, including block utilization, through the first quarter of the year.

Results of Reallocations

Once data for this period became available, managers reviewed the results of the reallocations from three perspectives: (a) impact (if any) on block utilization; (b) impact (if any) on overall capacity creation; and (c) response and continued support by stakeholders, including physicians, the OR staff, and senior leadership.

Impact on Block Utilization
The reallocation process yielded meaningful immediate improvement in the OR's overall block utilization. Overall block utilization in the inpatient suite—in which two departments swapped four-hour blocks—improved to 76 percent in Q1 2006 from 69 percent and 65 percent in Q3 and Q4 2005, respectively. Although several departments contributed to this improvement through modest utilization increases, the most significant gains were observed in *both* the department losing the four-hour block and the department gaining the four-hour block.

The results proved equally meaningful in the ambulatory suite, which achieved a block utilization rate of 70 percent in Q1 2006, up from 61 percent and 54 percent in Q3 and Q4 2005, respectively. In particular, the department losing a four-hour block doubled its utilization over one quarter, improving utilization from 30 percent to 60 percent—significantly closer to optimal levels.

Improvement in other efficiency metrics, such as turnaround time and first-case on-time start rates also indicated greater efficiency. Additionally, the short-term strategies that were implemented earlier, including extensions of select rooms, continued to show positive changes through Q1 2006.

Impact on Overall Capacity Creation
In addition to the internal efficiency benefits accrued to both inpatient and ambulatory OR suites, adapting the block schedule to actual demand also

increased OR capacity: In Q1 2006, the inpatient suite accommodated approximately 100 additional cases, and the ambulatory suite an additional 200 cases, compared to the previous quarter.

Response and Continued Support by Stakeholders

As the reallocation process continued to gain momentum, support increased from physicians, OR staff, and administrative stakeholders. Even representatives of departments that lost OR time supported the system's openness and objectivity. The OR staff also responded favorably, citing the benefits of working repeatedly with the same surgeons and an improved workload. Hospital leadership found that the new system reduced physician and OR staff complaints and appeared to hold longer-term promise of improved efficiency and profitability, and effective capacity creation.

In aggregate, much of the favorable response among the stakeholders was driven by the objectivity of the reallocation process, which allowed it to remain relatively apolitical. Rather than one individual making a set of subjective (or seemingly subjective) reallocation decisions, this process was guided by a consensus-driven policy, suggested by data, and implemented by a broad group of representatives.

Additional Questions and Considerations

Despite the improvements made to both OR scheduling efficiency and the process for maintaining it, further areas of opportunity remain. Memorial Hospital's ORs continue to face growth in surgical volume. Specific areas of future focus should involve:

- maintaining stakeholder support;
- continued review of the literature (and other evidence) regarding best practices with respect to OR scheduling and block scheduling specifically;
- continued evaluation of the reallocation process and its frequency;
- increased attention to utilization of staff and other resources; and
- an ongoing dialog with the hospital's strategic planners, so the OR scheduling system can reflect evolving hospital priorities.

Finally, while management and optimization of block utilization are critical to optimization of overall OR efficiency, to achieve maximum results, managers should continue to expand the evidence-based approach used in block scheduling to additional metrics relating to OR productivity and efficiency, and remain mindful of the dynamics among them.

Endnotes

1. Associations used or contacted included Association of OR Nurses (AORN), University Health Systems Consortium, American Association

of Clinical Directors, and the Health Care Advisory Board. Several search engines were used, including PubMed and ProQuest, and several journals were scanned directly, including *Harvard Business Review, Health Care Strategic Management, Health Care Management Review, OR Manager, AORN Journal*, and others.

2. Permanent members of the OR executive committee included the chief medical officer, chief operating officer, surgeon-in-chief, vice president of perioperative services, medical director of the ORs (anesthesiologist), and four chairs representing OR subcommittees (who also represented the largest services).

Reference

Patterson, P. A. 2004. "A Few Simple Rules for Managing Block Time in the Operating Room." [Online information accessed 2/20/09.] www.surgicaldirections.com/white_papers/OR%20Manager%20Block%20Time.pdf.

EVIDENCE-BASED CRITERIA FOR HOSPITAL EVACUATION: THE CASE OF HURRICANE KATRINA

K. Joanne McGlown, Stephen J. O'Connor, and Richard M. Shewchuk

Under most disaster scenarios, hospitals become places of refuge for the injured or sick. What happens when a major hospital itself is incapacitated and must be evacuated? (deBoisblanc 2005)

Hurricanes are the third most common cause for hospital evacuation. (Distefano et al. 2006)

Introduction

New Orleans...the "Big Easy"...the Crescent City...a city known for its jazz, incredible diversity of culinary delights, and "on the edge" lifestyles. Sitting below sea level on the Mississippi River, New Orleans is surrounded and protected by a series of levees and earthen dams. The infrastructure protecting the city has long been known to be vulnerable—a vulnerability that concerned engineers, city planners, and emergency management officials. However, many residents—and people in positions of authority—believed the city was blessed with good luck when it came to storms—that is, until August 2005.

Over the years there have been several near-miss hurricanes, but the last to strike the city with force was Betsy, in 1965. For the next 40 years, the area was hurricane-free, with storms veering to the west or east. This long history of being "storm-proof" provided a false sense of security when it came to hospital leaders' attention to disaster planning. But on Sunday, August 28, 2005, as Katrina mushroomed into a powerful Category 5 hurricane headed directly for New Orleans, the city's luck ran out.

The storm reached 1,000 miles across, with a predicted storm surge of up to 28 feet. Hundreds of thousands of Gulf Coast residents had evacuated, and an estimated 1 million people left the greater New Orleans area. On Monday, August 29, the eye of the storm passed just east of New Orleans, devastating the Mississippi Gulf Coast and creating one of the greatest natural disasters in U.S. history.

In the center of the below-sea-level "bowl" that was the city's heart sat the major medical centers, including the private, university-based Tulane University Hospital and Clinic (TUHC). TUHC lost power around 6:00 a.m. on Monday, and when several windows blew out, rain started to pour in. Yet, as morning broke, the city—and its hospitals—appeared to have withstood the storm with only moderate damage. President George W. Bush expressed thanks that New Orleans had "dodged the bullet" once again.

TUHC relocated its emergency department from its storm-safe location on the third floor back to ground level to see post-Katrina patients; internal facilities were relocated, and a tour of the building's exterior revealed an area severely wind damaged, but dry. In the aftermath of such a powerful storm, the hospital's situation appeared remarkably stable. But the sense of relief was short-lived.

At 9:30 p.m. the Hospital Command Center learned there was street flooding; water was rising approximately one inch every 10 to 15 minutes. Unable to receive confirmation as to the cause of the flooding, the emergency department and other critical departments were once again relocated to the third floor, and steps were taken to secure the physical plant. Hospital administrators were not aware that levees and floodwalls breached by the storm surge were allowing water to pour into the city, and that New Orleans was rapidly sinking into a third-world nightmare.

Soon electrical power, clean water, and communications capabilities were lost, crippling administrators' ability to provide critically needed services. The August heat was stifling. As backup generators failed, hospitals were thrust into darkness, temperatures soared, staff members worked in unbearable conditions, and critically ill patients rapidly deteriorated.

Kim Ryan, TUHC's chief operating officer (COO), had tracked the storm with her management team since Friday the 26th. The Command Center had been operational since Saturday. The team never considered the option of evacuating the hospital. Evacuation would put its tertiary and quaternary care patients at too great a physical risk; the plan had always been to "shelter in place" at TUHC, to hunker down until the threat was over. By 1:30 a.m. Tuesday morning, sheltering in place was increasingly untenable. Ryan awoke the CEO and the Hospital Corporation of America (HCA) regional director and, with their agreement, began feverishly to prioritize patients for evacuation. With no evacuation plan, and common-sense safe routes of ground evacuation no longer an option, Ryan's team began the Herculean task of throwing together an impromptu evacuation plan for some of the most critically ill patients in the city. How could the patients be evacuated, she wondered, and how did the situation ever deteriorate to this level?

Applying Evidence-Based Management

Step 1: Formulating the Research Question: What Do We Need to Know?

TUHC was a 362-bed university teaching hospital, a few years into a 99-year management agreement with HCA. Tulane had an active and nationally known emergency department and trauma program and provided a full range of the highest level of critical care and transplant services for adult and pediatric patients. As Katrina approached, between 30 and 40 TUHC patients were dependent on electrical equipment: ventilators, oscillators, and biventricular assist devices (500-pound pieces of equipment that could not be moved easily or safely).

The tragic situation Hurricane Katrina created for TUHC is the basis for the research question addressed in this case: *Did this hospital have an efficacious, systematic, and evidence-based plan for evacuation in the event of a disaster, and if so, what were the performance criteria for evacuation, and how were they applied?*

Internal and external hospital preparedness is an essential aspect of a hospital's emergency and disaster planning, but a task as difficult and dangerous as a full evacuation is an often neglected component. Many studies have described shortcomings in medical aspects of community emergency management plans, including confusion, lack of coordination, poor communication, lack of integrated planning, and inadequate training. At the hospital level, emergency planners face similar problems. In many parts of the country, the healthcare community's efforts to prepare for and respond to emergencies have been parochial and disjointed, with each facility or agency doing its own thing, often resulting in a breakdown in the delivery of medical care—a breach of faith with those who depend on these vital services.

Regional coordination among hospitals greatly assisted the evacuation of New Orleans–area patients and helped ensure continuity of care for thousands of people affected by the storm. The regionalization of hospitals began with federal Health Resources and Services Administration funding in 2002 and had fully matured prior to the landfall of Hurricane Katrina. However, issues still arose that should have been addressed years earlier:

- State officials lacked the authority to order replenishment of depleted supplies and arrange for patient evacuations when hospitals could no longer operate.
- An entity was needed to coordinate patient transportation.
- There was no system to track patients, and there was no way to know how many patients the region's hospitals could absorb, the acuity of those patients, and the resources they would need.

State and federal emergency planners and agencies had sounded alarms about New Orleans's precarious situation for years. As each hurricane season approached, geologists and climatologists warned of the potential devastating effects of a Category 3 or larger hurricane to the city. In 2002–2003, the Federal Emergency Management Agency sponsored a series of preparedness exercises implemented by the State of Louisiana Emergency Management Agency. The exercises were built around a hypothetical hurricane, called "Hurricane Pam," hitting New Orleans. The Hurricane Pam scenario was described by one physician as "so extreme that it was impossible to believe."

Work on this scenario continued in August 2004, and a few of the concepts of the working groups were implemented during Hurricane Katrina. The framework for a city emergency management plan had begun in New Orleans; planners assessed the local infrastructure, established coordination with the statewide hospital regionalization system, conducted city evacuation drills and planning, and addressed the need for attention to residents' psychosocial and personal issues. Yet, emergency planning and full integration across sectors at the city, parish, and state levels remained unfinished. One physician reported that hospital evacuation was not even addressed until the last stages of the Hurricane Pam exercise, and planning for it was incomplete when Hurricane Katrina landed.

In fact, a plethora of disaster plans existed for the New Orleans healthcare sector prior to Katrina, but to be useful they needed to be read, their implications understood, and their recommendations acted upon. Through the New Orleans Metropolitan Hospital Council, most hospitals, including TUHC, fully participated in the Hurricane Pam exercises.

Evacuation plans are widely acknowledged as something every hospital should have. The Joint Commission, the National Fire Protection Association through its Standard 1600, and state regulations require them. It is also a "priority" under the 2007 federal Department of Health and Human Services, Assistant Secretary for Preparedness Response funding programs; but there are no standards regarding what the plans should contain, nor are the basic competencies for hospital evacuation specified. Hospital executives decided not to acknowledge the worst-case scenario and, as Katrina approached, did not implement existing evacuation plans. In the end, the enormity of the disaster caught decision makers unprepared. They had not readied the processes and procedures that would have allowed them to respond appropriately.

This case examines the benefits of applying evidence-based practices to the environment of disaster management and the task of healthcare facility evacuation. Successful planning and response based on evidence offers many benefits: All hospitals would pay attention to the same critical issues and cease practices known to be harmful, reducing variability in preparedness and response, and they would adopt best practices. The question for

TUHC was: *Did this hospital have an evidence-based plan for evacuation in a disaster, and if so, what were the criteria and how were they used?*

Step 2: Acquiring the Evidence: How Do We Learn from Prior Disasters?

Research on disasters rarely achieves the rigor of randomized, double-blinded, clinical studies or even the less rigorous observational case-control or cohort studies. The evidence available in the disaster field is usually Level V research, the weakest type. That is, it relies on evidence-based opinions of respected authorities, descriptive studies, or reports of expert consensus committees. The limitations in these studies, often conducted under extreme conditions, are understandable since:

- most operational research on disaster medical planning has been conducted on sudden events, with no opportunity to develop a careful methodological strategy beforehand;
- most variables cannot be controlled;
- data collection generally must be retrospective, and over time, memories fade and recall bias becomes an issue;
- most disaster research uses qualitative methods and is heavily dependent on personal accounts and case studies;
- many research reports are not published in peer-reviewed journals; and
- early systematic studies have become dated and may provide unreliable advice regarding effective medical response.

Experts have recognized for some years that U.S. hospitals are inadequately prepared for disasters and that the evidence supporting critical decision areas, such as evacuation planning, is incomplete. In New Orleans, some evidence was disseminated to area planners and healthcare authorities, but it wasn't acted on.

At TUHC, the hospital's policy was to never evacuate, but to shelter in place for the protection of patients and staff. Planning never seriously addressed the worst-case scenario, and no contingency plans existed.

Hospitals are required to have a disaster plan and a type of hospital incident command system that is not only understood and implemented, but fully integrated with other systems in the community. The Joint Commission accreditation requirements and new federal guidelines for the National Integrated Management System may partially explain why almost all hospitals engage in community-wide emergency exercises and planning. Unfortunately, most drills and exercises are brief and include only staff on day shifts—clearly inadequate for actual emergencies, which can occur at any time of day or extend beyond a single shift. Emergency planners know that simply having a plan does not equal preparedness.

Locating evidence that would enable more adequate preparedness may be difficult for people with little understanding of the language of the disaster community. Nevertheless, information on hospital evacuation planning is available in federal, state, and local government documents and reports, legislation, and regulations; in scholarly articles; and from accreditation agencies, such as the Joint Commission.

Step 3: Assessing the Validity, Quality, and Applicability of the Evidence

Evacuations have historically been linked to high patient mortality because the process is stressful for acutely ill patients. However, when New Orleans hospitals were surrounded and then flooded with toxin-laden water, when they lost power and communications, when temperatures soared and sanitation deteriorated, the need to move all patients to a safer place became increasingly urgent.

Patients in certain clinical units faced greater-than-average risks. Infants in neonatal intensive care units require 1:1 clinical staff care, and those on life support had to be manually ventilated when the electricity failed. Transplant patients faced similar risks. Obese patients were especially difficult to move, and evacuating them was a challenge.

Many critically ill patients are attached (by relatively short tethers) to bulky, heavy, life-support equipment. But the air evacuation route required that patients—and their equipment—be transported to the rooftop. Carrying incapacitated patients *and* their equipment several floors up pitch-black stairwells in 100-plus degree temperatures was an extraordinary and exhausting feat; still, when other options ran out, it *was* successfully accomplished.

In Hurricane Katrina, the consequences of not using available information were horrific. The failure to translate existing knowledge into worthwhile and actionable processes resulted in a difficult evacuation process under the most miserable conditions, compounded by many difficulties that could have been avoided through improved planning and preparedness. Was the evidence presented or not? Did leaders engage in preparedness planning and simply fail to implement plans, or were the plans themselves inadequate?

By failing to plan for evacuation, the hospital lacked the adequate and appropriate resources to carry out an evacuation. Evacuations are labor-intensive under the best conditions, and the hospitals that were forced to evacuate had precious few staff members available to deliver critical patient care. The equipment and machinery required for a massive patient airlift, including aircraft, had not been prearranged.

The overarching responsibility of healthcare management leaders is to preserve the health, safety, and welfare of all patients, employees, and staff. The consequences of not being prepared can be death.

Barriers to Evacuation Planning

Extending research discoveries into public health and clinical practice is not easy. In New Orleans, barriers prevented hospitals from implementing evidence-based disaster planning. These barriers have been grouped as follows:

Type of Barrier	Primary Level of Operations
Macro-Environmental	Financial/System
Organizational/Structural	Trauma Center/Hospital
Professional/Personal	Individual Clinicians

Macro-environmental barriers can include financial, regulatory, and system factors that prevent a facility from implementing existing guidelines. **Structural** and **organizational barriers** arise because different providers make treatment decisions at different stages of care (such as in trauma care), and the potential for breakdowns in continuity of care exist at every boundary between units, disciplines, and departments. **Professional** and **personal barriers** include traditions, practice imperatives, styles of practice, and attitudes.

A number of barriers to hospital disaster planning efforts prior to Hurricane Katrina were identified either through the literature, personal interviews, or other sources:

- Planning was perceived as too cumbersome, chaotic, and confusing.
- There were too many plans by too many entities, and planning didn't involve or reach the right people, especially those at the top of the organization.
- There was a lack of leadership in implementing plans. The people most informed about the plan may have had too little authority within the hospital's hierarchy.
- Administrators may have viewed emergency and disaster planning as a costly endeavor, offering few benefits and marginal returns.
- Although a hospital is required by accrediting bodies or others to develop a disaster plan addressing facility evacuation, most administrators were not strongly motivated to support this effort, or they failed to believe a disaster event was likely to affect their hospital.
- Although there are standard measures of hospital preparedness, there are few standards for hospital evacuations.

Step 4: Applying the Evidence in Decision Making

When seeking to incorporate evidence-based planning into hospital evacuation plans, a hospital must overcome structural and organizational barriers and individual resistance. The literature suggests tackling these obstacles by:

1. Limiting the number of people in the evacuation planning process, ensuring that only relevant departments are represented;

2. Determining the resources needed in an evacuation, including transportation, and identifying other hospitals in the region that could receive patients or provide pharmaceuticals and supplies, negotiating agreements with them, and including them in exercises;
3. Assessing the location of various clinical units in the facility, with respect to logistical issues, should evacuation be necessary;
4. Developing protocols for evacuation implementation, specifying staff roles, and including a strategy for redeploying staff and remaining flexible to changes in units and their management, to maximize each employee's and unit's contribution to the evacuation; and
5. Framing implementation of evacuation as a research and learning opportunity.

Ryan, then COO and currently TUHC's CEO, reports that the hospital has "dramatically limited the number of people considered 'essential'" for disaster operations and staffing of the Command Center and that those who will be primary responders are "more knowledgeable of our planning at the department and facility levels." TUHC has taken to heart the recommendations in the literature, and the remaining steps listed above have already been implemented or are in process.

The primary responsibility for hospital emergency preparedness varies widely. A study of 1,750 U.S. hospitals found that the staff members most frequently designated by the CEO as the hospital's primary contact for emergency planning were located in various departments: security (24 percent), emergency services (17 percent), administration (13 percent), emergency management (12 percent), and facility operations or environmental services (10 percent) (Braun et al. 2006). Of these individuals, only 19 percent held positions classified as senior leadership. Most do not have easy or frequent access to the CEO.

When there is no single discipline or profession consistently responsible for hospital preparedness, and when senior executives are not routinely involved, emergency preparedness planning simply will not have sufficient resources or executive attention. Certainly, ensuring that high-level and challenging integrative emergency tasks are carried out, such as conducting a seamless evacuation effort, will be difficult. Both Jim Montgomery (then CEO) and Ryan report that having a "designated person at the facility to lead internal planning" is imperative and that preparedness has become a major priority for HCA CEOs since Katrina.

Step 5: Evaluating Results and Making Improvements

The evidence from post-action assessments identified opportunities for improvement of TUHC's preparedness for mass patient evacuation in the areas described below.

Current, Redundant, and Reliable Communication

Communication was the most critical factor in the determination to evacuate and the ease with which that process was completed. With landline phones inoperable, and when cell phones died, TUHC was unable to let the outside world know what was happening or plead for help. Clearly, newer technology and multiple, redundant systems should have been in place for both internal and external communication. The hospital has purchased a new satellite telephone system, with removable antenna, for the rooftop, as well as newer-generation satellite telephones and an 800 MHz radio system. A number of employees are ham radio operators, and the facility has purchased ham radio equipment to support the facility in future disasters.

Facility Evacuation Planning

TUHC developed a plan for total facility evacuation that is modifiable according to a storm's characteristics. Decisions will be made on the basis of the size of the storm, location of New Orleans within the "cone" of threat, and time to landfall. These plans are fully integrated with those of other area hospitals and include the triage and prioritization of patients, multiple transportation options, and staffing coverage for patients transferred to outside facilities.

Safety and Security of Facility

Like most hospitals, TUHC had a hospital security department that was trained, yet unarmed. The value of an armed security force became evident after Katrina, as looting and gunfire around the facility halted initial evacuation attempts. TUHC also recognizes the importance of staff members' sense of security in their decisions to remain on duty. However, management has not made developing a secure facility a higher priority.

Staffing and Processes for Patient Transfer and Routing

Internally, management reassessed staffing for emergencies. It now defines those who form the core "emergency team" as "A" responders. The backup team, called "B" responders, is the replacement team for the sleep cycle. A new "C" group of responders comprises nurses who will be dispersed to hospitals that will care for evacuated patients. Preplanning has identified facilities for receipt of evacuated patients, and staff will evacuate with them. In particular, they will care for patients on specialty equipment and neonates. Externally, major planning has been completed with peer HCA facilities. Each is aware of the types of patients they will receive and the staff that will be needed to care for them. In addition, TUHC fully supports the statewide system of bed tracking, coordinated by the state hospital association.

Equipment, Supplies, and Logistics for Mass Airlift and Patient Movement

Greater attention and planning have been given to food stores, water, and general supplies (central supply) as well as pharmaceutical stocks. HCA established a plan among all its hospitals at risk for hurricanes, providing coverage and resupply of critical stores. Agreements have been secured with 26 different helicopter services, through HCA Corporate, to ensure availability and access to aircraft for HCA patients, should airlift be required. Buses and drivers have been secured to bring employees to the facilities that will receive patients after evacuation. TUHC also was instrumental in leading initial discussions to preplan the mass evacuation of patients from the area, which would involve C-130 transport planes based at the Belle Chase Naval Air Station, near New Orleans.

Infrastructure Upgrades and Protection

TUHC's first-floor generator has been waterproofed, and sensors will warn of rising waters in the basement. An emergency generator was purchased for the second floor of the garage area, which is capable of operating one elevator for evacuations and providing air conditioning to the ICU. The hospital is digging a well, so that it has water should the city infrastructure fail again, and it has installed a backup fuel supply line in case fuel cannot be trucked in—an inevitability during a mandated citywide evacuation.

Improved Staff Training and Education

TUHC has participated in many drills and exercises with other local hospitals, organized through the Metropolitan Hospital Council and the state. This experience translates into continual education of all staff and employees to ensure familiarization with and preparedness for disaster response.

Interagency and Hospital Coordination

As stated earlier, New Orleans lacked a regional entity to coordinate patient transportation and tracking. The statewide hospital regionalization concept has been further strengthened, recognizing that hospital reporting and communication into a central, statewide command center were crucial aspects of patient flow and treatment during Katrina. In addition, the Metropolitan Hospital Council has remained active in integrating area hospitals through exercises and planning efforts.

Medical Records Information Sharing and Coordination

One serious issue faced by TUHC was the lack of an electronic medical records system, which would have enabled it to transfer patient information to receiving facilities or to a repository site safe from the storm. Medical records have since been restructured to allow remote access to critical patient information. A summary sheet of recent care delivery also can be generated on demand to accompany patients being evacuated.

Pet Care

TUHC, like many facilities in recent disasters, learned firsthand the importance of providing pet care for staff required to report to work in disasters. With no previous pet care experience, TUHC cared for more than 70 pets inside the facility until aid finally arrived. The hospital has since retained a veterinarian and staff who will care for its employees' pets. A bus and driver have also been reserved to evacuate the pets to a farm outside the city, where volunteers will help care for, feed, exercise, and provide companionship to the pets for as long as necessary.

Reimbursement Issues

The post-disaster impact on the reimbursement of care is a serious challenge faced by healthcare administrators. Katrina completely altered the demographic base of the city, and recovery efforts created additional financial hardships for those seeking medical care. Many lost jobs (and medical benefits) in the aftermath of Katrina, and the demand for medical beds in the future, are dependent on demographics.

Over the two years since Katrina, TUHC managers have revisited their experiences with the mass evacuation of patients in New Orleans. A few broad strategies have been identified as critical for successful implementation of hospital planning that also reflect what is needed in preparing for major disasters requiring patient evacuation (March 2006).

Suggested Strategy	TUHC's Response
1. Change the behavior of medical facility leadership	Involved medical staff more deeply in planning at the department and facility level. Developed a medical staff plan for response to any expected activity during a disaster.
2. Identify basic competencies to be addressed to ensure readiness for future evacuations	Identified competencies and skills required for patient triage, prioritization, and preparedness for evacuation. Identified processes for preparing and packaging

(Continued)

2. Identify basic competencies to be addressed to ensure readiness for future evacuations *(Continued)*	patients for safe evacuation. Added these topics to orientation of new employees and continuing education of existing staff. Included same in exercises for nursing, medical, and ancillary staff.
3. Prepare the organization for behavioral change in disaster response and recovery	HCA identified required system changes, with a plan for "cultural change" throughout the corporate structure. Modifications included systematic change and processes required to establish interoperability of planning and functions among all facilities, and development of a support network for the transport and care of patients when facility evacuation is required.
4. Explore the question: "Is the way we did it really the best way?"	Post-event assessments examined every action taken, decision made, and outcome. Detailed timelines reflect all issues and management problems faced and decisions made. Working through and with other healthcare facilities, the city's Metropolitan Hospital Council, and HCA partner facilities, decisions were critiqued and formed the basis for revisions to disaster plans and enhancement of facility and community policies and procedures for hospital evacuation.
5. Establish a comprehensive and tailored education process to enhance employee preparedness for and education on evacuation	TUHC has fully incorporated this topic into new and existing employee education. Exercises reflect revised plans and procedures that address processes for patient evacuation, and citywide exercises allow process improvement for this eventuality.

6. Organize for continuous improvement	All actions reflect a newfound commitment by TUHC and HCA to improvement and assessment of actions in the area of patient evacuation.

All changes described above have resulted in enhancements to TUHC's emergency and disaster plans and have effected corporate policy changes throughout the HCA network.

Conclusion

The U.S. healthcare system is said to be isolated in its planning activities and is possibly the weakest link in emergency response. There may be no way to avert another Katrina. Mother Nature does as she wishes. But in healthcare facility evacuation, our challenge is to implement strong mitigation efforts to protect structures and encourage preparedness planning at the personal, family, and institutional levels.

In reference to the profession of emergency management, Pfeffer and Sutton (2006) describe evidence-based management as "a way of thinking about what you and your organization know and what you don't know, what is working and isn't, and what to try next." They go on to say that in the field of emergency and disaster management, as in general management, the "demands for decisions are relentless, information is incomplete, and even the very best executives make many mistakes and face constant criticism and second-guessing from insiders and outsiders." Evidence-based management can't improve every managerial decision and action; however, there are effective steps presented here that can create the right mind-set.

Two years after Katrina, Ryan is vigilant in ensuring that her facility is prepared for the next disaster. TUHC failed to benefit from evidence that existed at the time of Katrina, but it will benefit in future disasters from the hard lessons learned. Its analyses and subsequent actions have added to the knowledge base about hospital evacuations and survivability under the direst conditions.

References

Braun, I. B., N. V. Wineman, N. L. Finn, J. A. Barbera, S. P. Schmaltz, and J. M. Loeb. 2006. "Integrating Hospitals into Community Emergency Preparedness Planning." *Annals of Internal Medicine* 144 (11): 799–811.

deBoisblanc, B. P. 2005. "Black Hawk, Please Come Down: Reflections on a Hospital's Struggle to Survive in the Wake of Hurricane Katrina." *American Journal of Respiratory and Critical Care Medicine* 172: 1239–40.

Distefano, S. M., J. M. Graf, A. W. Lowry, and G. C. Sitler. 2006. "Getting Kids From the Big Easy Hospitals to Our Place (Not Easy): Preparing, Improvising, and Caring for Children During Mass Transport After a Disaster." *Pediatrics* 117: S421–27.

March, A. 2006. *Facilitating Implementation of Evidence-Based Guidelines in Hospital Settings: Learning from Trauma Centers. Publication No. 930.* New York: The Commonwealth Fund.

Pfeffer, J., and R. I. Sutton. 2006. "Profiting from Evidence-Based Management." *Strategy and Leadership* 34: 35–42.

IMPROVING THE HEALTH STATUS OF UNDERSERVED CHILDREN IN HOUSTON'S EAST END

Patricia Gail Bray

Introduction

During the past decade, evidence-based medicine has inspired the development of evidence-based management in healthcare, but to date, few healthcare organizations use this technique. Moreover, there are no reports of health foundations that rely on an EB management approach to guide improvements in community health status or even their own funding decisions. Although commentators suggest that charitable foundations are uniquely placed to promote evidence-based policy, health foundations in Texas typically use the judgments of program officers rather than the analyses of trained researchers to guide their grant-making decisions.

Houston-based St. Luke's Episcopal Health System created a grant-making public charity in 1997.[1] The foundation's mission is to enhance community health for the underserved, not only through its grants, but also through a public health research agenda that includes a comprehensive assessment and evaluation of the community's health. In short, St. Luke's Episcopal Health Charities was set up to integrate philanthropy with community-based research through an EB management approach. This approach includes a commitment to adopt a culture that values management research, trains managers in the use of research for decision making, and diffuses research techniques and results throughout the organization. This case study will highlight how The Charities used an EB management approach to conduct community-based research and fund healthcare interventions in an underserved neighborhood of Houston.

Following a model similar to that advanced by the Center for Health Management Research, the Charities's leadership began by working side by side with the University of Texas School of Public Health. The leaders soon realized that they had a prime opportunity to bridge public health theory with public health practice for the purpose of advancing community health. Embracing a public health research orientation meant focus-

TABLE 19.1
Decision-
Making Models
Contrasted

Model Type	Initial Steps	Research Steps	Action Steps	Evaluation Steps
Population Health Model	Analyze health issues	Set priorities	Take action	Evaluate results
St. Luke's Research Model	• Site selection • Data collection, with community participation	In collaboration with the community: • Set strategic priorities • Build consensus	• Intervention design • Build capacity	Evaluate results
Evidence-Based Management Model	Frame the question	Acquire information (evidence) and assess its • validity • quality • applicability	• Present the evidence • Apply it to the decision	Evaluate results

ing on improving health status at a population, rather than an individual, level. The population health model for assessment includes four steps: analysis of health issues, priority setting, taking action, and evaluating results. (Although this model was not explicitly connected to evidence-based management at the time, the Public Health Agency of Canada [2007] now links a population health approach to evidence-based decision making.)

Building on this simple framework, we expanded the model in two ways (see Table 19.1):

- *Community involvement.* By focusing the work on a particular neighborhood, we hoped to engage multiple community partners to assist in decision making and priority setting.
- *Action component.* Our action component included both intervention and capacity building, to improve prospects for sustainability.

The Charities's hybrid model uses mixed research methods, which align remarkably well with decision-making features of the EB management model developed by John Hsu and colleagues (2006). Their model was developed as a "toolbox" for healthcare managers and policymakers. For this chapter, we adopt the six decision-making steps that constitute the toolbox and examine how a similar model was put into practice at the Charities. In practice, the steps of these models are not always performed in a linear fashion. Not only is there significant overlap between steps, but there also can be non-sequential movement between them.

Applying Evidence-Based Management

Step 1: Framing the Research Question

Setting the Context

The first step in the EB management process is to frame the research question in a way that captures relevant elements of the proposed intervention, desired outcome, setting, time frame, and population of concern. For the Charities, these elements could be specifically defined. Because of our mission, the intervention needed to be directed at health, and the leadership team adopted the World Health Organization's well-known definition of *health* as "a state of complete physical, mental, and social well-being and not merely the absence of disease or infirmity." Thus, we included social, cultural, economic, and environmental health indicators in our research. The desired outcome was to assess community healthcare needs comprehensively, so that the Charities could fund interventions that would have the best chance of enhancing residents' overall health.

The time frame of the proposed intervention was the current fiscal year, since funding allocations are distributed annually. The population, specified by our mission, included underserved families and children, primarily those living below the federal poverty level. The board of directors and the leadership team then narrowed the study population specifically to children—a priority group for funding. As a result, we framed the following research question: *How do we best assess the health status of children in an underserved neighborhood in Houston?*

Since a large city like Houston has many underserved neighborhoods, the leadership team wanted to select the one with the highest proportion of underserved children. This step generated the question: *How do we identify, prioritize, and select underserved communities?* The choice of the study area could be based on conventional wisdom, since the most underserved neighborhoods are usually common knowledge. Or a study area could be chosen on the basis of formal or informal connections to nonprofit organizations or the advice of board members and staff. Or it could be chosen based on anecdotal knowledge from local foundations working on similar interventions. However, the Charities's intention, since its founding, was to fund interventions in areas of greatest need, *as determined by research*. Ultimately, both types of evidence—colloquial and research-based—guided site selection.

In step one of the Charities's model, the leadership team needed to acquire preliminary evidence to choose an appropriate neighborhood. This evidence included best-practice knowledge from the literature, meta-analysis of recent local studies, and a broad review of recent and appropriate secondary data.

For this study, the individual team members were all trained in public health and had experience working in underserved communities to improve health status. Due to this unique team composition, there was a strong academic connection, as well as a community connection. Pulling together an inventory of recent research regarding Houston neighborhoods and children was relatively straightforward for this team, and existing relationships with local health departments and advocacy agencies facilitated our initial research.

The Meta-Analysis

We conducted a meta-analysis of six major needs assessments conducted in or around the Houston area during the early to mid 1990s. Three of the six were released in 1997, so the team had current data regarding most traditional maternal and child health indicators, including:

- Distribution of births and birth rates
- Births to mothers aged 17 and under
- Unmarried mothers under age 18
- Late or no prenatal care
- Low birth weight
- Infant deaths
- Infant mortality rate and
- Death rate for children aged 1 to 14

Three retrospective studies from the mid-1990s that assessed the quality of life for Houston-area children enabled the team to document significant overall progress in maternal and child health over the previous decade, but pockets of concern remained. Specifically, the infant mortality rate for all ethnicities except African Americans had dropped below the Healthy People 2000 objective of no more than 7 deaths per 1,000 live births. The percentage of mothers seeking prenatal care in the first trimester had increased overall, but fell well short of the objective among Hispanic and African-American mothers and especially among teenage mothers of all ethnicities. The low-birth-weight rate had remained relatively constant since 1990, but rates of low-birth-weight babies among African American and teenage mothers remained higher than among other groups.

As of the late 1990s, health problems appeared to have shifted from infants to children and adolescents. It appeared that, as children grew older, they were increasingly at risk for preventable problems, such as unintentional injuries, homicide, suicide, substance abuse, child abuse and neglect, developmental problems, and lead poisoning. (Unintentional injury was the leading cause of death.) These findings were critical for the team selecting the research site.

Additionally, the data indicated that 21 percent of Houston-area children lived in poverty. This figure was increasing, along with the proportion of children who were Medicaid eligible. The high school dropout rate was rising, as was the percentage of teens not in school or working. On the basis of this evidence, the team determined to place more focus on prevention, ameliorating problems related to social disadvantage and social problems in general. Therefore, choosing a neighborhood experiencing these kinds of challenges among youth was critical.

These criteria narrowed the search to several underserved neighborhoods, including Houston's East End, a predominantly Hispanic neighborhood where a significant proportion of the population lived in poverty. The East End contains three distinct neighborhoods and approximately 50,000 residents. A majority of the area's 16,000 children are uninsured and live below 200 percent of the federal poverty level. Since the mission of the Charities is to serve the underserved, and the funding priorities were to be geared toward children, evidence gathered so far indicated this geographic area fit our criteria well. Next we had to obtain data that would help us understand this specific study area better.

Step 2: Acquiring the Relevant Information

Obtaining Secondary Data at the Neighborhood Level

At this point, we refined our research question to: *What evidence exists about the current health status of children in Houston's East End neighborhood?* Sub-county data are usually difficult to obtain, but essential when assessing how to improve neighborhood health status in a very large county such as Harris County, which has a population larger than 24 U.S. states. The Charities employed a combination of epidemiological, statistical, and estimation methods to create a comprehensive array of data. We collected some primary data, particularly through cluster sampling, and relevant secondary data from the U.S. Census Bureau and Texas Department of State Health Services, among others. Demographic statistics were collected and included race/ethnicity, age distribution, median income, poverty level, education, and number of single-parent households. We looked at traditional maternal and child health indicators, along with other data available from birth certificates, such as mothers' education—an important predictor of child well-being and a good example of how much variance can be found at the sub-county level. Approximately 36 percent of all mothers in Harris County did not have a high school education, whereas in Houston's East End, 63 percent of mothers did not. Data on environmental conditions, such as air, water, and land quality, were obtained from the Environmental Protection Agency.

Most of these sub-county data were geo-coded and put on the Charities's website (www.slehc.org), using an interactive mapping program. This effort made them available for use by other foundations, health planners, and community-based organizations.

Obtaining Qualitative Data

One way we involved the community in the project was to engage members in developing qualitative data through multiple methods, including a community-based participatory research (CBPR) approach (Agency for Healthcare Research and Quality and W.K. Kellogg Foundation 2001). During the mid-1990s, articles in the health assessment literature began to suggest that researchers should expand their traditional approach to assessing, funding, and evaluating healthcare needs and begin to include the voice of the community. The Charities's leadership team was similarly interested in understanding local needs from the community's perspective, believing that community members' perceptions mattered just as much as the reality framed by the researchers. Over time, the core of our neighborhood-level assessment model has evolved to emphasize the community voice throughout the research process. It helped validate our planning process and refine research results by identifying areas for intervention and providing a focus for our research.

Use of participatory, qualitative research techniques, performed in partnership with the University of Texas, allowed community members to identify and analyze the major issues of concern, from their point of view. CBPR, which is gaining more and more of a research following, is a semi-structured process of learning from and with people rapidly and progressively, face to face, in a relaxed manner and in an informal setting. It encourages self-reflection, analysis, questioning, and learning. This study asked questions of community participants, such as:

- Are some age groups of greater concern than others?
- What are the major issues by age group?
- What is the relative importance of each issue?
- What factors have produced these issues in the community?
- How might these issues be addressed?
- What community resources might be directed to help?
- Could resources from outside the community be helpful?

This study helped fill in missing gaps from the earlier evidence. Here we see an example of the nonlinearity of the Charities's model: By investigating community needs (and gathering more evidence) with a qualitative approach, the participants were also able to assess the accuracy of the earlier evidence. In summary, after all of the evidence was collected, the team was able to identify the children most at risk in the East End and the children with the severest problems. We also had a good understanding of what those problems entailed. Without the multimethod approach, we would not have been alerted, for example, to rising gang membership among teenage Hispanic girls.

Steps 3 and 4: Assessing and Presenting the Evidence

How can we corroborate what we learned in the previous step? This step is important for anyone employing an EB management approach, but it is crucial for leaders working in philanthropy and public health. There is a general tendency to rely on expert evidence in both areas, but the consequences of doing so can lead to funding interventions that are ineffective and inefficient. Relying solely on one type of evidence—colloquial, anecdotal, or just secondary data—may prompt funding of interventions that do not fit the community or are not sustainable. Because the community's perceptions of need often differ dramatically from what the experts think, the evidence should be verified in partnership with community members.

In this case, if we had based our decisions solely on the secondary data, we would have made key mistakes in funding interventions. For example, we learned that childhood asthma rates were increasing in Houston, an impression corroborated by data issued by the Centers for Disease Control and Prevention. Interventions to curb this kind of problem are usually complex, costly, and long term. However, our leadership team discovered during the qualitative phase of the study that, in a certain elementary school in the East End, children were being given Benadryl during the school day to treat their asthma symptoms. Consequently, they were sleepy in class, which led to other complications. When all of the evidence—colloquial and research based—was considered, we selected a simple intervention to solve this immediate problem. A mobile unit delivering primary care would be parked at the school one day per week, providing children access to asthma care and appropriate medication.

Limitations of the Evidence

There are likely to be limitations to the data that decision makers have, no matter how they were collected. The following checklist asks key questions for assessing data accuracy.

Quantitative Data Checklist

- Are the research findings valid?
- Does the evidence provide a complete and balanced viewpoint?
- Is the analysis appropriate?
- Is the source credible?

Qualitative Data Checklist

- Is the context of the study adequately described?
- Are the sample selection and data collection processes appropriate?
- Is the analysis appropriate?
- Are the findings valid?

Such questions need to be asked, even when the data come from credible sources such as the U.S. Census Bureau and the Texas Department of State Health Services. Census data are, after all, derived from a survey, which means these data suffer from all of the challenges associated with survey data, such as sampling error and selection bias. Additionally, since the complete census data set is updated only every decade, it can become outdated and decreasingly useful, especially at the neighborhood level or in rapidly changing locales. State-collected vital statistics are subject to inaccuracies in information provided by respondents. For example, mortality statistics are based on death certificates, which often do not accurately record important comorbidities for decedents with chronic diseases, such as diabetes. Further, good data on illnesses and risk factors—including smoking prevalence, drug and alcohol use, overweight and obesity rates, mental illnesses, and oral health—are difficult to obtain at the sub-county level. These data also come primarily from surveys and are subject to the limitations noted above.

Yet, we found that many questions about data accuracy could be answered by community members—that is, residents and community-based organization leaders living and working in the East End. We could not feasibly ask every individual in the East End to participate, so we developed a sampling matrix to identify the major sectors of the community that should be represented in our research. As with any qualitative study, the sample size was limited. To overcome any bias in the results, we made the sample broad, seeking the perspective of representatives of all sectors of the community.

Community Sampling Matrix by Sectors		
Political	Economic	Health
Police	Communication	Recreational
Other community groups	Individuals	Education
Religious	Social welfare	Immigration and refugee support

While community members could not validate the research findings and the evidence gathered from secondary data, they could corroborate qualitative findings with knowledge gleaned from other community-based studies. For example, in most underserved communities, despite the ethnic diversity, we see common needs, such as mental health and dental services and access to primary care. Additionally, community members could at least comment on the findings and the assessment of needs and resources for their community. Most important, community members could *prioritize* those needs.

The Charities's leadership team convened a neighborhood task force to review our findings and comment on the accuracy of the information. Including the community in this process helped during all the remaining steps of the model.

Assessing the Applicability of the Evidence

Most of the data collected (both quantitative and qualitative) were focused on this particular geographic community. However, they were not always applicable for our purposes. For example, the data pointed strongly to the need to eradicate poverty in the East End—a worthy recommendation, but not one that is possible with the Charities's limited resources. To ensure applicability of the data, the Charities's leadership team formed, from the larger neighborhood task force, a formal, more focused collaboration called the East End Healthy Children's Collaborative, which nine years later remains an organized, informal group.

The Collaborative went through a formal strategic prioritization process to select a few gaps in child health on which to focus the intervention: primary healthcare, mental health, dental health, and child care. The evidence collected and the prioritized recommendations were shared with the broader community via a formal, written report. At this point, the EB management model clearly aligned with the model we adopted, completing the strategic priority-setting and consensus-building steps before initiating the action steps. And we had answered the questions in the checklist featured in the next section.

In addition to our own interventions, we initiated a funding collaborative so that multiple foundations could focus their efforts more effectively on this neighborhood. The result was a deep commitment by the public health community, funding agencies, and East End stakeholders to work together to enhance the health status of the entire community. For example, the qualitative research revealed two areas of need that were not addressed immediately by the East End Collaborative: domestic violence and teen gangs. Since the collaboration facilitated by the Charities had not selected these issues, it recommended them to other foundations as immediate concerns worthy of funding.

Step 5: Assessing the Actionability of the Evidence and Applying It to Decisions

Once the quantitative and qualitative data had been collected, verified, and reviewed for applicability, the next step was to determine whether the recommendations could be implemented in the designated time frame. Typically, there are more needs than resources, and interventions must be identified as short term or long term. However, if the processes above have been successful, and the recommendations prioritized, time-relevant programs can be proposed for funding.

The decision making involved in defining interventions is critical. The first question in the following checklist asks whether there is information on what needs to be done. There may be several best practice methods to choose from for a specified intervention, and some best practices may fit better than others for a particular neighborhood. Sometimes, no best-practice models fit a proposed intervention. For example, during the study in the East End, we learned that elementary students as young as nine years old were thinking about suicide. During a key informant interview, a school district official told us that a regional psychologist was assigned to various elementary schools in the East End area to address this concern. The East End Collaborative agreed that a licensed professional counselor should be put on the mobile primary care unit that was currently serving several elementary schools. This innovative solution was proposed to the Charities, and the board of directors subsequently approved the grant. Within the first few months of the intervention, the regional psychologist was no longer needed in schools served by the mobile unit.

Checklist for Actionability of the Evidence
• Is there information on what needs to be done?
• Is there information on how to do it?
• Is there information on how to monitor whether it is working?

The final step in the EB management model we used requires an evaluation of possible decision options. Is there adequate evidence to make a sound decision? Is more than one option available? The experience of our work in the East End tells us that there are usually multiple options, and once again, we relied on the community voice to guide the prioritization of options. Community-based organizations have firsthand experience and can usually discern which options will work better under different circumstances.

Having adequate, up-to-date information is always a challenge in public health research. For example, mental health needs in children are pervasive, yet we do not have adequate baseline information at the sub-county level. The Office of the U.S. Surgeon General (1999) has reported that 20 percent of all children aged 9 to 17 "have some kind of mental health problem" and that 5 percent of those with a problem develop a serious emotional disturbance. But the beauty of using mixed research methods is that hidden needs are uncovered, as are innovative solutions to resolving those needs. So, even if adequate information about how to resolve a particular problem is not available—especially a newly discovered one, such as teens' finding new substances to abuse—decisions nevertheless can be made that may improve community health status, directly and indirectly.

Checklist for Adequacy of the Evidence
• What are the decision options?
• Do I have a complete list of options?
• What does the available credible evidence indicate about each of the decision options?

- Is there a dominant option? More than one option involving trade-offs?
- Are there uncertain options, or is there inadequate information?

Step 6: Evaluating Results

A key question in this step asks whether there is a method to determine whether the intervention is working. Evaluation metrics must be selected before the intervention is implemented, so that progress can be measured at regular intervals and so that program experience does not bias the choice of measures. To obtain aggregate data for all funded programs, the Charities developed standard outcome measures for use by all grantee organizations. Standardization is a good way to monitor progress, and if multiple agencies are delivering a similar service in the community, their outcomes can be aggregated for a different level of analysis and possible identification of new best-practice models.

For philanthropic and public health organizations interested in funding interventions and achieving outcomes to enhance child health status, taking an EB management approach can be more effective and sustainable than ad hoc and less-well-informed methods. As mentioned earlier, there are always more health needs than resources, due to systemic problems such as poverty and barriers related to undocumented immigrants. With an EB management approach that includes community voice, the health foundation can be more in tune with the community's perceived needs. Findings can be organized to serve as a systematic, credible resource for other stakeholders, foundations, and nonprofits with the same goal of enhancing the health status of the community. Additional local, state, and federal funding can help local nonprofits that use the evidence. In the East End, for example, a small nonprofit clinic used our data in its application to become a federally qualified health center, which resulted in an influx of significant federal funding and more holistic health services for the underserved.

Additional outputs and outcomes included substantial enhancements in the following eight areas:

- Primary care
- Children's Health Insurance Program (CHIP)/Medicaid
- Designation as a federally qualified health center
- Youth development
- Mental health
- Dental health
- Child care
- Fitness and nutrition

These improvements have had dramatic positive effects on the health of neighborhood residents, including reductions in the rate of preventable problems. Enhancements to primary care and mental health services came about through the funding of mobile clinics that provide thousands of children with access to care, free or low-cost pharmaceuticals, and immunizations. The project enrolled virtually all eligible East End children (approximately 15,000) in either CHIP or Medicaid, increasing access to care, establishing a medical home for them, and decreasing their use of the public hospital's emergency department for routine care. Dental health services were added, and since the designation of the federally qualified health center, dental services and mental health services are permanently provided in the East End.

With the creation of a new "children's corridor," child care services were increased so that East End parents could take advantage of enhanced social services, including general education development and English as a second language classes, nutrition classes, and fitness opportunities. Tennis courts, a new gymnasium, soccer fields, and baseball fields are under construction. In one obesity prevention program for children, 68 percent of participants improved their body mass index, and 53 percent of children and families report healthier eating habits.

The Charities's total funding for the nine years of programming since the beginning of the Houston East End research is $5.5 million. Our widely shared research has enabled many more foundations to invest significant resources in this underserved community. The result is a dramatic improvement in individual and community health status and better programs and systems.

Conclusion and Challenges

Many groups benefited from the EB management approach taken by the Charities to enhance health status in an underserved community, including:

- The children and families who live there
- Nonprofit providers in the community
- Local funders interested in improving health status
- State and national funders interested in funding local health interventions
- Local researchers
- Undergraduate and graduate school interns
- City and county health departments
- Public health clinics
- Mental health clinics
- Dental health clinics
- Private and public emergency departments and
- The Charities, as an effective grant maker

The Charities's evidence-based model is one that has been tested and implemented in ten neighborhoods in the Houston area and one in

Austin. While the challenges may be different for each underserved community, our experience indicates that the evidence-based approach can lead to stronger, more relevant programming to improve community health. In addition, this approach encourages organization leaders to value research, train managers in the use of research, and diffuse research methods and findings throughout their organizations. We believe it is an effective decision-making method for health foundations and public health agencies interested in improving population health status and community outcomes.

Endnote

1. Unlike most new health foundations created in the past two decades, this public charity is not a "conversion foundation" (that is, one formed from the sale or change of a nonprofit organization—typically a hospital or health insurance plan—to a for-profit organization).

References

Agency for Healthcare Research and Quality and W. K. Kellogg Foundation. 2001. "Community-Based Participatory Research: Conference Summary." [Online information; retrieved 2/23/09.] www.ahrq.gov/about/cpcr/cbpr.

Hsu, J., L. Arroyo, I. Graetz, E. Neuwirth, J. Schmittdiel, T. G. Rundall, and M. Gibson. 2006. *Methods for Developing Actionable Evidence for Consumers of Health Services Research (Match Study): A Report from Organizational Decision-Maker Discussion Groups & A Toolbox for Making Informed Decisions.* #290-00-0015. Rockville, MD.: Agency for Healthcare Research and Quality.

Public Health Agency of Canada. 2007. *What is the Population Health Approach?* Ottawa, Ontario: Public Health Agency of Canada.

U.S. Surgeon General. 1999. *Surgeon General's Report on Mental Health.* Washington, DC: U.S. Department of Health and Human Services.

LESSONS LEARNED, AND WHERE DO WE GO FROM HERE?

SUMMING UP AND LESSONS LEARNED

Commentary by Richard D'Aquila, David J. Fine, and Anthony R. Kovner

Based on interviews conducted, condensed, and edited by Anthony R. Kovner.

What Is the Message of This Book?

D'Aquila: The principal message is that management decisions, initiatives, and programs should be grounded in a process whereby managers ask the right questions and assemble the right information for the decision. It seems like a simple and logical way to make important decisions, but it is not universally practiced, with the result that managers make many faulty decisions. But even managers who attempt to base their actions on evidence can always make decisions better and continuously improve the process.

Fine: One of the reasons the U.S. hospital sector performs relatively poorly is that its managers are part of a culture based on institutional subjectivism, in which they do not make decisions based on a careful review of evidence and objective criteria. These are important decisions, too, and range across resource allocation, marketing, and quality. In this book we present 14 cases and case situations where managers have tried to make decisions based on the reported literature on comparable situations and other relevant studies. Some of these case studies aren't "home runs" but initial attempts to use a process similar to that of EB management. If more managers would make this kind of effort in their organizations, the industry could move toward a baseline of vastly improved hospital performance.

For example, in Houston, every small suburban hospital is trying to launch an open-heart [coronary artery bypass graft surgery—CABG] program, including 100-bed hospitals with low volume. They would be doing 50 to 75 cases per year. Every bit of the reported literature says that much higher volume is needed to have high quality. But in Houston, where we're unregulated, they are free to do it. What needs to happen, given our free market, is for someone who buys that service commercially—say, Aetna—to refuse to pay for a CABG unless the hospital performs at least 250 cases a year. We are trying to get this message across to practicing hospitals and insurance executives and employers. Basically, a large employer shouldn't want managers to be making decisions in any way other than by using EB management, or a similar, research-based process.

Kovner: Large amounts of resources are allocated in healthcare organizations based on managerial decisions. EB management builds on evidence-based medicine, which argues that to the extent possible, medical interventions should be made only when they result in positive, predictable outcomes. We assume that the quality of managerial decision making can be greatly improved if managers have available to them more of the existing evidence relevant to making an important decision. Part of high-quality decision making is a deliberative process that is transparent and in which important points of view are represented. The EB management process is, admittedly, more likely to result in a set of outcomes involving options, each with trade-offs, rather than an identification of a one-best-way solution, but our working hypothesis is that it will nonetheless result in better decisions.

Implementing EB management requires a culture shift in organizations that many managers are not willing to lead. Part of this shift starts with the manager, who must admit to not having all the answers and who must know where all the important evidence lies; listen to all points of view among significant stakeholders; and understand that management interventions must be framed as questions that are answerable. A cultural context facilitating evidence-based decision making, to include an effective deliberative process, is not common. Most healthcare CEOs believe that management research is the job of universities, foundations, and government, and not a managerial responsibility.

Why Don't More Managers Adopt an Evidence-Based Approach?

D'Aquila: I've spent 20 years thinking about how decisions are made. As a consultant, this was what we were doing. At the start we would assemble some quick data to tease out the bad decisions. Then we would use data, dashboards, and evidence. This book says that managers have to invest more time in having an open mind, framing the right questions, using high-quality data, and interpreting it correctly.

Fine: EB management is a foreign language. It's as simple as that. If managers were comfortable reading and interpreting the published literature they would do so. But they've never been prepared for it. For a number of years, I've been close to several medical schools. Most undergraduate medical school curricula have a required course on how to read and use the published literature. This is not a course to organize and conduct studies, but to interpret studies. In the AUPHA-accredited healthcare management programs, we give students six to nine credit hours of how to do rudimentary statistics and some quantitative methods that barely take them to the level of novice. The goal should be to help managers learn how to read someone else's work and see whether it's germane to what they are trying to do. So, in the field of management, unlike clinical medicine, students are not taught to value and depend on studies as physicians are and, in part because of this lower priority, there are fewer studies done.

Kovner: All managers use evidence—however flawed—to make decisions. But most managers and consultants are not rewarded for basing their interventions on the best available evidence. EB management is not widely used primarily for three reasons. First, the business case for return on investment has not yet been reliably made for EB management. Second, widespread use of EB management would shift power away from senior managers toward junior managers armed with capability and will to obtain higher-quality evidence. Third, governing boards do not regularly review the quality of the managerial decision-making process (nor is this reviewed by external parties) as to available information obtained or the nature of the deliberative process.

What Did We Learn While Writing This Book?

D'Aquila: Wolfman and Strauman wrote their case studies in institutions where I have worked, where we obtained exceptional but usable data, constructed good predictive models based on accurate data, and field-tested them to make sure they worked. These models have stood the test of time. They have proved reliable and valid and have provided good going-forward mechanisms for doing what they intended to do. At Weill-Cornell, we went back to the surgeons, shrank their block time, and increased utilization. At Yale-New Haven, the bed model was accurate for our projections in making bed capacity and other changes. This book validated for me what I had been doing all along and what we have been doing these past two years at Yale-New Haven.

Fine: I have become much better informed about what people have written over the last decade. From a practitioner's viewpoint, I knew something was missing, and that was reports on what has been going on around the country in EB management. The core of this book will be very helpful to practitioners. Describing a process such as EB management creates a structure within which managers can experiment. James A. Hamilton published a book like this in 1960, which proposed a 14-step problem-solving process, starting with "Define the problem by apprehending the real issues of the situation and stating the problem precisely," and ending with "Implement action to carry out the selected solution." In a way, this was a precursor to what we're doing here. But Hamilton wasn't widely followed. My hope is that we have produced a book documenting such a substantial practitioner outlook and perspective, with fairly lengthy examples across a wide range of topics, that many managers will be inspired to give EB management a try.

Kovner: I learned that a key step in EB management is "framing the question." This includes starting with the management challenge, such as reducing long waits in the emergency department (ED), then reframing it as a set of research questions focusing on ED design, primary care delivery in the ED, and bed control. Another key step in EB management is a high-quality deliberative process. This includes having a manager responsible and accountable for seeing to it that balanced viewpoints are at the table and that available evidence is generated and effectively arrayed. This manager tracks all major decisions that must be made and identifies the supporting evidence for them. After the fact, the manager reviews a sample of interventions to consider whether the process can be improved going forward.

What Are Our Plans for Further Developing EB Management in Our Organization and Professional Career?

D'Aquila: At YNHH we have eight major service lines—heart, cancer, pediatrics, neurosciences, transplant, psychiatry, women's health, and ambulatory—plus traditional hospital support. Each service line leader has the same job description and is responsible for more than a half-dozen critical issues: patient satisfaction, employee and physician satisfaction, quality, regulatory readiness, patient flow and throughput, business plan development, and volume targets. They also are responsible for the service line's profit and loss (few hospitals can actually produce a profit and loss statement for a cardiac service line that makes sense at the doctor, procedure, and patient levels). Typically, service line managers make bad decisions if they do not have incentives to grow revenues. They turn away two cases because this will take them over the expense budget, but these cases may bring in four times the revenue for twice the expense.

Operations support functions as a total consulting firm. We have four team leaders, a couple of clericals, and 10 percent of the time of 40 to 50 Six Sigma green belts who work in other areas. This costs us now $400,000 a year. We use an entry-level manager and an administrative fellow, too. This year we'll probably double the cost and size of the operation, as we did this initially on a shoestring. Here's an example of how we used operations support: To reduce nurse overtime, I hired one of our team leaders as a consultant, for $10,000 a month. Our database on overtime was after the fact, and overtime reports were put in the hands of our managers 15 to 20 days after closing. Now system nurse managers have overtime data on a desk-top for daily review. This concurrent review process has resulted in massive behavior change. We sent them to school, gave them a class on financial fundamentals for first-line managers. Before, no one had ever taught them how to manage overtime and do appropriate daily staffing, or what kinds of systems and reports were available to them. No one had ever taught them strategies to reduce overtime. Now we require authorization of overtime based on volume incentives. Now we offer more overtime to nurses who haven't reached their weekly maximum [before offering to nurses who have reached their maximum, which would cost more]. We've saved $10 million a year on this.

For my first year's budget, I started with an authorized budget that had $8 million for the bottom line, and we delivered $20 million on the bottom line. Revenues were up $14 million, and expenses were under by $7 million. I hit the budget ball out of the park. We financed operations support through cost reductions, risk avoidance, and revenue enhancement. All the things I've done over the years had to be accomplished through the back door. Here, I've had free rein to do what I want. I've been able to "just do it." At YNHH, we have 8,000 employees. We've just given all of them a full 3 percent bonus check in addition to their raises. Our pay-for-performance was tied to patient satisfaction and financial targets. Nothing is more exciting than to give your employees this kind of bonus compensation.

Managers can't manage successfully in our oppressive hospital reimbursement environment unless we factor evidence into our decisions and actions. There are four areas of high-performance management in hospitals: (1) quality—which means your hospital is in the top 2 to 3 percent nationally on all major indicators and that it scores consistently in the 90+ percentile; (2) extremely high patient satisfaction—which means improving your patient satisfaction scores faster than everyone else; (3) margin—your hospital must be strategic, be profitable, replenish its resources, and invest in the future; growth has to be strategic, for if you get the "wrong" volume this clobbers you financially; and (4) be the employer of choice—this involves benefits, employee recognition, health and wellness, how employees feel about where they work, communication with supervisors and the leadership team, and employee development, recruitment, and retention. All four areas involve all kinds of decisions and choices—thousands of them—that need to be based on the best available evidence. Leadership is delivering these outcomes, focusing on the right things.

Fine: I'm becoming increasingly strident about this. I'm really challenging executives at St. Luke's to "show me the beef." The chief nursing officer is making demands as to how she wants to increase her nurse staffing. On instinct, I would say she is right. Competitive considerations say she is right. The California legislature–mandated nurse staffing ratios say she is right. We're trying to pose the research question and measure the results, taking half the units and moving them to the more costly model, and then we'll see if it makes any difference for patient outcomes and nursing satisfaction. So we'll spend $5 million rather than $10 million and see whether the new staffing ratios work.

Another example concerns our five new suburban facilities. How large should these be? Where is the literature that can inform our decisions as to optimal operating size? Also, we have in our system now two comfortable business units and one that is struggling, holding on, just, to budgeted performance. We have a tremendous need to compare this unit to other organizations with similar case-mix indices (ours is over 2.0). Finally, after jawboning for a year, we've gotten people to understand that they must find metrics with which to create reasonable comparisons. That hasn't been the style around here.

Kovner: I plan to work toward establishing the Center for Evidence-Based Management at NYU/Wagner and to consult with a large health system to implement EB management. NYU/Wagner is a large school of public affairs in New York City, where many faculty and students are already engaged in teaching and researching EB management. The new center would have three parts: teaching, research, and support. The Teaching Division would offer a two-year master's of science degree in management, which is currently available, with a concentration on EB management. Much of the curriculum is already in place and new courses would be developed specifically for this program. The master's would be largely delivered online, with four to six weeks of residence in New York City, over 65 to 70 weeks, for cohorts of 25 students going to school half-time. Tuition would be paid principally by employers.

The Research Division would carry out five to ten research initiatives each year. This would include original research and meta-analyses. The Research Division would also conduct, on a fee-for-service basis, searches and analyses of the literature and the Web on management topics. The Research Division would be funded by annual contributions with three-year commitments by health and other large nonprofit and government systems. The Support Division would supply management and marketing for the Teaching and Research Divisions. Support for the Center for Evidence-Based Management would be sought from organizations participating in the teaching and research programs and from philanthropy and government. A board composed of representatives from the participating systems and others would guide and advise the Center.

As a consultant, I would focus on working with a large health system's top management team of 40 to 50 individuals. I would examine the current process for making management decisions, to include interviewing current managers as to how the present system works and should work to become more evidence-based. I would lead the effort along with a top manager designated by the CEO to champion this project. That individual's responsibilities would include developing and managing an electronic bulletin board on which major management decisions are tracked. New rules would be established regarding the process of decision making (without slowing that process down). Rules would include thresholds for decisions to be included in the tracking process, methods for generating searches, and deliberating on evidence obtained. Managers would be trained in the EB management decision-making process. There would be sample hindsight review of major decisions already taken to see how the process can be improved. Finally, development of and competency in EB management would be formally measured as part of management's performance review and included in compensation decisions.

Reference

Hamilton, J. A. 1960. *Decision Making in Hospital Administration and Medical Care: A Casebook*. Minneapolis: University of Minnesota Press.

APPENDIX A: SELECTED SOURCES OF INFORMATION ON THE EVIDENCE-BASED APPROACH AND RELATED TOPICS

Sara Mody

This concise reference includes many of the best sources available on evidence-based management and represents the insights of the field's leading researchers. While the literature discussing EB management has grown in the past several years, the practice is still in its infancy.

The list of resources has multiple audiences. First, we hope that students of healthcare management will view the sources on the evidence-based approach as a start for further study. Second, educators will find resources to facilitate teaching students the skills needed to execute EB management in their future organizations. Third, managers of health systems will find practical information to help develop their skills for implementing an evidence-based approach to decision making. Fourth, those wishing to perform management research will see the resources available to help fund and guide their role in furthering the use of and the research contributing to the evidence-based approach. The section concludes with a list of websites for further research and potential funding sources. In summary, the five parts are:

- The Evidence-Based Approach
- Teaching Evidence-Based Management
- Implications of Evidence-Based Management for Managers
- Doing Evidence-Based Management Research
- Web-Based Resources

"Must read" sources are starred (★).

Print Resources

Trends in Evidence-Based Management

Evidence-based movements in other industries: Industries other than healthcare have incorporated evidence-based approaches into their cultures. Evidence-based initiatives have begun in conservation, crime prevention, education, government, librarianship, medicine, nursing, social work, software engineering, sports, and others.

Looking internationally for guidance: The United Kingdom and Canada are leaders in EB management. Government-supported organizations, such as the Canadian Health Services Research Foundation and the NHS National Library for Health, exist with the goal of furthering an evidence-based practice in both medicine and management. United States healthcare students, managers, and researchers can begin to rely more on international evidence as support for local initiatives.

Integration of EB management into healthcare graduate education: Educators have begun to incorporate the skills for EB management into their courses. Literature discussions have occurred to debate the best way to include the ideas of EB management in graduate programs.

Increasing accountability by the public and hospital boards demanded: As the public gains greater access to healthcare quality and management data and as boards place increasing emphasis on outcomes, managers and administrators will be held more accountable for the consequences of their decisions. Increased accountability will lead to a greater demand of evidence-based decision-making.

Increased research focus on quality, accessibility, and efficiency: Concerns of measuring and maintaining quality of care have become a top research topic as more and more hospital data become publicly available. Accessibility and efficiency have also become pressing topics as the United States struggles to deliver better care to more people without exponential growth in costs. Below is a summary of the research topics from some of the leading organizations.

- Advisory Board Company: business strategy, operations, and general management issues
- Agency for Healthcare Research and Quality (AHRQ): improving outcomes, quality, cost, use, and accessibility of healthcare, concentrating on safety and quality, efficiency, effectiveness, and organizational excellence
- Center for Health Management Research (CHMR): clinical integration and decision support, performance measurement and reporting systems, managing care, and managing quality
- Canadian Health Services Research Foundation (CHSRF): managing for quality and safety, managing the healthcare workplace, primary healthcare, nursing leadership, organization, and policy
- Health Research and Educational Trust (HRET): community health, coverage and access, and quality and safety
- Accelerating Change and Transformation in Organizations and Networks (ACTION): quality and safety; pay-for-performance and performance measurement; quality improvement for diverse populations; strengthening of the healthcare safety net, structure, organization, management, and financing of the health system; and management of chronic illness

The Evidence-Based Approach

Booth, A. 2006. "Clear and Present Questions: Formulating Questions for Evidence Based Practice." *Library Hi Tech* 24 (3): 355–368.

The article offers a solid foundation for understanding the importance of question formulation. Booth provides a conceptual framework for formulating an answerable research question. The SPICE model considers all the following factors when creating a question: Setting—where? Perspective—for whom? Intervention—what? Comparison—compared with what? Evaluation—with what result? His discussion calls the reader's attention to the difficulty of framing questions while emphasizing the impact question design can have on the resulting research. Through the article, Booth begins to bridge the literature gap between evidence-based healthcare and evidence-based practices in other fields.

★ Gray, J. A. M. 2001. *Evidence-Based Healthcare: How to Make Health Policy and Management Decisions*. 2nd ed. Edinburgh, Scotland: Churchill Livingstone.

Gray presents an explanation of the evidence-based approach with a unique perspective as he draws on his experiences during a career in public health in the United Kingdom. Chapters 1 through 3 detail the history of healthcare, identifying the root causes leading up to and supporting an evidence-based approach. Gray further explains the complex nature of the healthcare decisions before leading the reader through the evidence-based approach in chapters 4 through 6. Gray also offers specific guides for healthcare management in chapters 7 and 9, where he explains developing a culture that supports evidence-based decisions and developing individual skills for managing evidence. Chapters 8 and 10 provide guides for evidence-based public health and consulting. The appendices offer tactics for finding, filtering, appraising, and storing evidence. The book is well written and entertaining to read. Gray provides clear definitions, key concepts, illustrative stories, analytical frameworks, implementation guides, and anecdotal evidence.

★ Hsu, J., L. Arroyo, I. Graetz, E. Neuwirth, J. Schmittdiel, T. G. Rundall, and M. Gibson. 2006. *Methods for Developing Actionable Evidence for Consumers of Health Services Research (Match Study): A Report from Organizational Decision-Maker Discussion Groups & A Toolbox for Making Informed Decisions*. Publication No. 290-00-0015. Rockville, MD: U.S. Agency for Healthcare Research and Quality.

Truly one of a kind—Hsu et al. designed this study and publication to help managers. The authors created an implementation methodology called the Informed Decisions Toolbox. The toolbox breaks the evidence-based approach into six steps: framing the question behind the decision, finding sources of information, assessing the accuracy of the information, assessing the applicability of the information, assessing the actionability of the information, and determining if you have adequate information. In the spirit of the evidence-based approach, the authors created the toolbox based on interviews with senior health service managers, and then refined the toolbox after piloting the approach with six Sutter Health managers. The authors also make recommendations for researchers, encouraging them to more closely align their work with the decisions managers make in addition to advising them to take steps to make findings more accessible to decision makers.

Kovner, A. R., J. Elton, and J. Billings. 2000. "Evidence-Based Management." *Frontiers of Health Services Management* **16 (4): 3–26.**

The authors succinctly walk the reader through the environment supporting EB management, the current position of management research, and the approaches that parallel EB management. The authors define EB management as a committed use of empirical evidence while also considering best practices and ideas. According to the authors, successful organizations will have a questioning culture that remains dedicated to making decisions on the best evidence available. A culture that includes systematic documentation and assessment of decisions will further support evidence-based decision making. Additionally, the authors recommend the creation of EB management cooperatives to bring together managers, consultants, and researchers to share information. Four vignettes support the authors' view that the evidence-based approach serves as a beneficial long-run investment. The article provides a good base for understanding the present state of EB management and where it may go in the future.

★ Kovner, A. R. and T. G. Rundall. 2006. "Evidence-based Management Reconsidered." *Frontiers of Health Services Management* **22 (3): 3–21.**

The article serves as a brief overview and resource guide by providing resources for health services research and guidelines for framing the question, presenting the evidence, and building a questioning culture. The authors emphasize that managers should understand the limitations of research—specifically, that evidence will never provide an unquestionable solution. Instead, evidence will enlighten decision making, allowing managers to better understand the problems and consequences of their decisions, increase stakeholder communication, and foster creative decision making. Managers will have the most success looking to evidence for help in answering questions regarding core business transactions, operational management, and strategic management. Furthermore, the authors offer four suggestions for increasing the use of evidence; ultimately though, understanding and addressing organizational and personal barriers will lead to better acceptance and use of evidence.

Learmonth, M. 2006. "Is There Such a Thing as 'Evidence-Based Management?': A Commentary on Rousseau's 2005 Presidential Address." *Academy of Management Review* **31 (4): 1089–1091.**

Learmonth argues that there are two problems with Rousseau's endorsement of EB management. First, management researchers consistently debate what counts as legitimate evidence. Learmonth worries that the lack of consensus among researchers will inevitably lead to more ambiguity in decision making. Second, EB management presents the possibility that some evidence may be disregarded in order to frame an issue to support a decision maker's opinion rather than being used to present a balanced argument.

★ Pfeffer, J., and R. Sutton. 2006. *Hard Facts, Dangerous Half-Truths and Total Nonsense: Profiting from Evidence-based Management.* **Boston: Harvard Business School Press.**

Pfeffer and Sutton see EB management as having two defined characteristics. First, EB management requires the willingness to ignore previously held beliefs and conventional wisdom when making decisions, and, instead, necessitates acting only on well-supported facts. Second, managers using the evidence-based approach should show unwavering dedication to finding the information needed to make more informed decisions. In the book, the authors identify barriers to implementing an evidence-based approach and outline seven principles to help companies overcome these obstacles. Unlike other books, the authors provide details of other decision-making models and explain why they are often confused with the evidence-based approach. The authors pose thought-provoking questions and support their perspectives with evidence, anecdotes, and humor.

Rousseau, D. M. 2006. "Is There Such a Thing as 'Evidence-Based Management'?" *Academy of Management Review* **31 (2): 256–269.**

Rousseau's 2005 presidential address for the annual meeting of the Academy of Management brings our attention to the common managerial practice of making decisions based on personal experience, consultants' recommendations, or weak evidence. Even if the evidence is available, many managers see using evidence as a threat to their decision-making power. EB management in practice involves integrating the best evidence available with manager expertise or client/customer preference. Rousseau outlines the characteristics of an evidence-based practice: learning about cause-effect relationships; identifying variations that affect outcomes; fostering a culture that practices evidence-based decision making and participates in research; participating in information sharing; creating decision support systems; and supporting access to organizational knowledge. Rousseau also discusses the insufficient support for EB management in management education, which does not have the curriculum to teach students to use evidence in decisions.

————. 2006. "Keeping an Open Mind About Evidence-Based Management: A Reply to Learmonth's Commentary." *Academy of Management Review* 31 (4): 1091–1093.

Rousseau agrees that management research lacks consensus but feels that a movement toward EB management will encourage more consistent research findings. Furthermore, Rousseau sees Learmonth's concerns of politics to really be concerns that qualitative evidence may not hold up to the standards EB management may come to use and that the validity of qualitative evidence will be diminished due to misuse. Most important, Learmonth and Rousseau agree that while EB management has great potential, a debate among all parties involved needs to occur to see the theory come to fruition.

★ Rundall, T. G., P. F. Martelli, L. Arroyo, R. McCurdy, I. Graetz, E. B. Neuwirth, P. Curtis, J. Schmittdiel, M. Gibson, and J. Hsu. 2007. "The Informed Decisions Toolbox: Tools for Knowledge Transfer and Performance Improvement." *Journal of Healthcare Management* 52 (5): 325–340.

The article provides a review of many key articles in this list. The authors cover the history of EB management, give advice to aid in the effective use of the EB management process, and discuss four leader-driven strategies for building an organization that supports EB management. Highlights from the Hsu Toolbox are included in the appendix.

Shortell, S. M., T. G. Rundall, and J. Hsu. 2007. "Improving Patient Care by Linking Evidence-based Medicine and Evidence-based Management." *The Journal of the American Medical Association* 298 (6): 673–676.

The authors state the key to reliable, long-term improvement in the quality of the U.S. healthcare system lies in linking evidence-based medicine to EB management. Evidence-based medicine defines treatment patterns while EB management focuses on organizational issues affecting the delivery of care. The authors offer four solutions for promoting the integration of evidence-based medicine and EB management: synthesizing EB management research, expanding EB management research networks, fostering a market for integration, and educating healthcare professionals in the use of evidence-based medicine and EB management.

Walshe, K., and T. G. Rundall. 2001. "Evidence-Based Management: From Theory to Practice in Healthcare." *The Milbank Quarterly* 79 (3): 429–57.

The article presents a thorough academic overview of EB management without being overwhelming. The authors explain how the rise of evidence-based medicine resulted in questions of how healthcare managers make their decisions—specifically, the role they allow evidence to play. While management encourages clinicians to adopt an evidence-based approach, they have yet to strongly adopt a similar method to their managerial decisions. Evidence-based medicine and EB management have similar problems—the overuse of ineffective solutions, the misuse of viable solutions, and the underuse of effective solutions; however, differences in culture, research base, and the decision-making process make the practice of EB management unique. Additionally, Walshe and Rundall use their experiences at the Center for Health Management Research to explore building relationships between researchers and managers that foster the use of evidence.

Teaching Evidence-Based Management

To help students practice EB management in their future careers, their graduate education should encourage the development of the following six skills. The resources listed provide background for developing each skill.

Skill 1: Using Critical Thinking

★ The Foundation and Center for Critical Thinking: www.critical thinking.org/index.cfm

The center hopes to enhance the level of teaching at all education levels by focusing on "assessment, research, instructional strategies, Socratic questioning, critical reading and writing, higher order thinking, quality enhancement, and competency standards" in addition to offering opportunities for professional development. The website is well laid out and easy to navigate, with links to articles that discuss critical thinking and its fundamental concepts. The center has resources for background information regarding issues in the area of critical thinking and developing a "questioning mind."

Moore, B., and R. Parker. 2003. *Critical Thinking*. 7th ed. New York: McGraw-Hill. Online Learning Center. [Online information; retrieved 2/20/07.], highered.mcgraw-hill.com/sites/0072818816/ information_center_view0/.

The authors break the concept of critical thinking into three parts. The first section provides an introduction to critical thinking. The second part addresses "Rhetorical Ploys and Common Fallacies." The book concludes with a discussion of deductive, inductive, and causal arguments. Students should walk away with the ability to distinguish supported and unsupported claims. The entire book and instructor's manual are available online. The student online version provides overviews, objectives, quizzes, flash cards, frequently asked questions, application advice, and Powerpoint tutorials for each chapter.

Skill 2: Using a Library

★ Association of College & Research Libraries. 2007. "Information Literacy Competency Standards for Higher Education." [Online article; retrieved 1/29/07.] www.ala.org/ala/acrl/acrlstandards/informationliteracycompetency.htm.

The article provides an overview of information literacy and its influence in promoting lifelong learning. In addition, the authors discuss information literacy in regards to information technology, higher education, and pedagogy. The document's key features are the detailed analysis of each competency broken into standards, performance indicators, and outcomes.

New York University (NYU) Libraries. 1999. "New York University Libraries Information Literacy Competencies Statement." [Online information; retrieved 1/29/07.] library.nyu.edu/research/health/tutorial/competencies.htm.

The article provides a concise and adapted version of the standards from the Association of College & Research Libraries by describing nine competencies NYU students should have to be information literate. The article breaks each competency into a few demonstrable skills. According to the document, the competencies require an understanding of the information needed, scholarly process, organization of information, information sources, accessing information, evaluating information, synthesizing information, information and society, and information and lifelong learning.

Skill 3: Recognizing Valid and Reliable Statistics and Understanding Applicability of Evidence

The *Journal of the American Medical Association* (*JAMA*) sponsored a series called "The User's Guides to the Medical Literature," compiled and published by the Evidence-Based Medicine Working Group. Some of the most applicable articles for managers are:

Drummond, M. F., W. S. Richardson, B. J. O'Brien, M. Levine, and D. Heyland. 1997. "Users' Guides to the Medical Literature. XIII. How to Use an Article on Economic Analysis of Clinical Practice." *The Journal of the American Medical Association* 277(19): 1552–7

Evidence-Based Medicine Resource Center. 2007. "The Evidence-Based Medicine Resource Center Bibliography." [Online information; retrieved 2/7/07.] www.ebmny.org/ebmbib.html.

Compiled by Patricia E. Gallagher, AHIP, the listed sources guide the reader to sources that help increase his or her understanding and use of quantitative analysis, medical and clinical journals, systematic reviews, research methods, and statistics. The author also references sources that provide advice on getting evidence into practice.

Giacomini, M. K., and D. J. Cook. 2000. "Users' Guides to the Medical Literature: XXIII. Qualitative Research in Healthcare." *The Journal of the American Medical Association* 284: 357-62.

Richardson, W. S., and A. S. Detsky. 1995. "Users' Guides to the Medical Literature. VII. How to Use a Clinical Decision Analysis." *The Journal of the American Medical Association.* 273: 1292–5.

Skill 4: Knowing What to Do When the Evidence Is Insufficient or Conflicting

★ Canadian Health Services Research Foundation (CHSRF). 2006. "Keys: Knowledge Exchange and the Production of Research." [Online information; retrieved 1/29/07.] www.chsrf.ca/keys/production_e.php.

This part of the CHSRF website provides "keys" for knowledge transfer and exchange. The information walks the reader through the research process, including what needs to be done before starting research, when starting research, and during research.

Skill 5: Understanding Healthcare Organizations and Process

★ Griffith, J., and K. White. 2006. *The Well-Managed Healthcare Organization.* 6th ed. Chicago: Health Administration Press.

This comprehensive guide to managing healthcare organizations covers increasing patient volume to enhancing quality of care to maintaining the physical plant. The book also addresses the role of preventive and non-acute services and stresses the value of the continuum of care. Decisions discussed support the evidence-based approach. The authors break chapters into discussion around one concept in terms of function, organization and personnel, measurement and information systems, and the managerial role. Each chapter concludes with suggestions for further readings.

★ Kovner, A. and J. R. Knickman (eds.). 2008. *Jonas & Kovner's Healthcare Delivery in the United States*. 9th ed. New York: Springer Publishing Company.

The book presents a discussion of top academics and practitioners regarding the major issues in healthcare delivery. A review of the basics of the healthcare industry and the provision of care leads into a conversation about the drivers affecting change within the industry. In addition to health services delivery, the book touches on health policy and public health issues as well. The authors break the topic into four parts: perspectives, providing healthcare, system performance, and futures.

Kovner, A. R., and D. Neuhauser (eds.). 2004. *Health Services Management: Readings, Cases and Commentary*. 8th ed. Chicago: Health Administration Press.

This book moves healthcare issues from theory to practice. The authors organized the perspectives of academics and practitioners around the following topics: the role of the manager, control, organizational design, professional integration, and adaptation. Cases then illustrate topics in settings like a faculty practice, a community health center, rural hospitals, and HMOs.

Skill 6: Teaching Evidence-Based Management

Fine, D. 2006. "Toward the Evolution of a Newly Skilled Managerial Class for Healthcare Organizations." *Frontiers of Health Services Management* 22 (3): 31–35.

Fine discusses the changing environment of healthcare management. No longer can managers rely on "gut" decisions or depend on an industrial engineering department to consider the evidence for them. For success, organizations need questioning cultures led by managers with the ability to analyze and use available information.

Rousseau, D. M., and S. McCarthy. 2007. "Evidence-Based Management: Educating Managers From an Evidence-Based Perspective." *Academy of Management Learning and Education* 6 (1): 84–101.

Drawing from other fields, Rousseau and McCarthy summarize six principles of evidence-based teaching. The paper outlines the current barriers to teaching an evidence-based approach to management students. In addition, the authors support relationships between researchers and teachers to further the acceptance of EB management.

Welton, W., L. Reed, and A. Kovner (eds.). 2003. "Teaching Evidence-based Healthcare Management." *The Journal of Health Administration Education* **20 (4): 221–329.**

This special edition includes articles that address the challenges of teaching an evidence-based and market-relevant approach to healthcare management. The contributors address different facets of and solutions to this challenge. Griffith suggests higher standards and the measurement of teaching outcomes. Kovner highlights the importance of narratives in learning the evidence-based approach. Finkler looks at teaching future financial managers how to use evidence. Rundall considers making doctoral programs more focused on evidence. Mick addresses the development of faculty, especially their influence in promoting a research culture. Bradley proposes competency teaching as a solution for when there is not enough evidence to link measurable competencies to job performance. Arndt and Bigelow provide guidance for the future of healthcare management education programs. Schlichting explores creating and circulating evidence in a large, academic healthcare system.

Implications of Evidence-Based Management for Managers

EB management has three main implications for managers. They will need to capitalize on the evidence and knowledge within their own organizations, understand that evidence-based decision-making ultimately leads to evidence-based implementation, and change the culture of their organizations to support evidence-based decisions. The sources below provide a starting point for further development.

Association of State and Territorial Health Officials. 2005. "Knowledge Management for Public Health Professionals." [Online article; retrieved 2/7/07.] www.astho.org/pubs/ASTHO-Knowledge-Management.pdf.

The Association of State and Territorial Health Officials, who support the creation and implementation of policies and programs for the states' public health departments, supported this publication. The document provides guidance for knowledge management agendas in state departments. The article introduces basic knowledge management concepts and describes how these work in a public health context, concluding with recommendations for implementation.

Canadian Health Services Research Foundation. "Is Research Working for You?" Ottawa, Ontario, n.d.

CHSRF has designed a tool to help organizations determine their capability to "acquire, assess, adapt, and apply research." The tool aims to help organizations discover strengths and identify weaknesses. To request a copy of the self-assessment, please contact research.use@chsrf.ca.

★ Davenport, T. H., and L. Prusak. 2000. *Working Knowledge: How Organizations Manage What They Know*. 2nd ed. Boston: Harvard Business School Press.

Many organizations fail to realize they can find the knowledge they seek within their own walls. More often than not, the resources are simply inaccessible. Davenport and Prusak, both consultants, candidly put forward their experiences working with more than 30 companies grappling with the intricacies of knowledge management. They separate the ideas of data, information, and knowledge while discussing the importance of knowledge management for a firm's overall success. Instead of developing a defined system for knowledge management, the authors highlight key issues and applicable ideas to help companies harness their experience and expertise.

Harvey, G., A. Oftus-Hills, J. Rycroft-Malon, A. Titchen, A. Kitson, B. McCormack, and K. Seers. 2002. "Getting Evidence Into Practice: The Role and Function of Facilitation." *Journal of Advanced Nursing* 37 (6): 577–588.

Harvey et al., using the concept analysis approach, recommend the development of a facilitator role to help move ideas from evidence to practice. Based on a research literature and influential texts, the authors state that the facilitator should "help and enable rather than tell or persuade," with his or her focus split between achieving project goals, developing individuals' skills, and improving the process of implementing evidence-based ideas. Overall, the article starts defining the role of the facilitator, but the authors feel further research will help delineate the varying models of facilitation in use.

Kovner, A. R. 2005. "Factors Associated with Use of Management Research by Health Systems." (Working paper.) Chicago: Center for Health Management Research.

Kovner performed research to evaluate knowledge transfer between researchers and managers involved with the Center for Health Management Research. Through 64 telephone interviews with health system managers, knowledge transfer was examined in four areas: diabetes management programs, budgeting and strategic priorities, performance indicators, and incentive compensation. The paper clearly presents its findings alongside strategies to improve the use of EB management principles.

Mack, K. E., M. A. Crawford, and M. C. Reed. 2004. *Decision Making for Improved Performance.* **Chicago: Health Administration Press.**

Managers will find this a great book to use for an implementation guide. Mack, Crawford, and Reed create a seven-step approach that will help lead to better decisions. The method centers on the idea that all decisions should help the organization meet its mission and maintain its financial well-being. To solidify the concept for the readers, the authors conclude with an illustrative case study examining the use of the seven steps in a hospital. The authors include practice materials, tools, guides, and checklists.

Nutley, S., H. Davies, and I. Walter. 2003. *Evidence-Based Policy and Practice: Cross Sector Lessons From the UK.* **(Keynote paper for the Social Policy Research and Evaluation Conference, Wellington, UK.)**

The paper provides an experience-supported discussion of implementing the use of evidence. The authors discuss their experience in encouraging evidence-based policy and practice in the United Kingdom. The lessons they learned from promoting the use of evidence are understanding what counts as evidence, developing a strategic approach to the creation of evidence, using effective dissemination avenues to ensure wide access to knowledge, and beginning initiatives to ensure policy uses available evidence. The appendices provide reviews of key insights such as a cross-sector review of evidence-based movements, improving dissemination, and types of research utilization.

★ **Stewart, R. 2002.** *Evidence-based Management: A Practical Guide for Health Professionals.* **Oxford: Radcliffe Medical Press.**

Stewart creates a guide demonstrating how to apply the principles of evidence-based medicine to managerial decision making. The book suggests methods of evaluating performance and discusses common obstacles with recommendations to overcome them. Overall, the book offers a concise overview of EB management and how to put the principle into practice.

Examples of Healthcare Organizations Using an Evidence-Based Approach

Canadian Healthcare System
www.canadian-healthcare.org

Group Health Cooperative Health System (Seattle, WA)
www.ghc.org

Henry Ford Health System (Detroit, MI)
www.henryfordhealth.org

Intermountain Healthcare (Salt Lake City, UT)
intermountainhealthcare.org/xp/public

Kaiser Permanente
www.kaiserpermanente.org

National Health Service
www.nhs.uk

Park Nicollet Health Services (Minneapolis, MN)
www.parknicollet.com

Sentara Healthcare (Norfolk, VA)
www.sentara.com/sentara

Sharp HealthCare (San Diego, CA)
www.sharp.com

Spectrum Health (West Michigan)
www.spectrum-health.org

Sutter Health (Sacramento, CA)
www.sutterhealth.org

Department of Veterans Affairs Health Care
www1.va.gov/health

Virginia Mason Medical Center (Seattle, WA)
www.virginiamason.org

Doing Evidence-Based Management Research

The resources below should help guide those wishing to perform management research. Successful research projects require a unique relationship between the researchers and decision makers. Some examples of EB management research have also been provided for reference.

Conducting Research

Alexander, J. A., L. R. Herald, H. J. Jiang, and I. Fraser. 2007. "Increasing the Relevance of Research to Healthcare Managers: Hospital CEO Imperatives for Improving Quality and Lowering Costs." *Healthcare Management Review* 32 (2): 150–159.

The article helps guide the EB management research agenda and researchers' approach to health services research. The authors conducted a series of semistructured interviews with a convenience sample of hospital and system leaders focusing on present and future challenges regarding quality, costs, and efficiency in addition to potential solutions. The interviews highlighted the importance of researchers taking a proactive role in getting their research into the hands of potential users and using those users to shape future research.

Denzin, N. K., and Y. S. Lincoln (eds.). 2005. *Handbook of Qualitative Research*. 3rd ed. Thousand Oaks, CA: Sage Publications.

This book provides a thorough overview of qualitative research. The editors have divided the subject into the following sections for discussion: Locating the Field; Paradigms and Perspectives in Contention; Strategies of Inquirers; Methods of Collecting and Analyzing Empirical Materials; The Art and Practice of Interpretation, Evaluation, and Presentation; and The Future of Qualitative Research. Made up of contributions from the top academics in human sciences, it is no wonder the book is considered to be the authority of qualitative research.

Drummond, M. F., G. L. Stoddart, and G. W. Torrance. 2005. *Methods for the Economic Evaluation of Healthcare Programmes*. 3rd ed. Oxford: Oxford University Press.

Drummond, Stoddart, and Torrance provide an outline of the methodology of economic analysis in addition to a generalized critical appraisal list for use with any study. Cost analysis, cost-effectiveness analysis, cost-utility analysis, and cost-benefit analysis are all covered. The authors also provide instruction on collecting data and presenting an economic analysis to decision makers.

Sox, H. C., M. A. Blatt, M. C. Higgins, and K. I. Marton. 2006. *Medical Decision Making*. Philadelphia, PA: The American College of Physicians.

This book leads the reader through the medical decision process. In general, this entails determining the probability of outcomes, gauging the accuracy of clinical data, and evaluating new information in order to make decisions about patient care. The authors use clinical examples to illustrate concepts. Each chapter concludes with self-assessment questions. In addition, the authors provide an annotated bibliography for further exploration of the literature on medical decision making.

Fostering Partnerships Between Researchers and Decision Makers

★ Canadian Health Services Research Foundation. 2007. "Productive Partnerships: Report on the 2002 CHRSF Annual Invitational Workshop." [Online information; retrieved 2/6/07.] www.chsrf .ca/knowledge_transfer/pdf/2002_workshop_report_e.pdf.

Based on feedback from the participants of the Annual Invitational Workshop in 2002, the paper assesses partnerships between researchers and decision makers. The paper attempts to define successful partnerships, explain the benefits of partnering, and provide tips for creating successful relationships. In summary, access to applicable research and fostering long-term and productive relationships appear to be the main benefits of partnering. Furthermore, in order for a relationship to remain beneficial, the following conditions must occur: cultural sensitivity, trust, commitment, clear roles and expectations, partnership with the entire organization, and organizational support.

Lavis, L. N., D. Robertson, J. M. Woodside, C. McLeod, and J. Abelson. 2003. "How Can Research Organizations More Effectively Transfer Research Knowledge to Decision Makers?" *The Milbank Quarterly* 18 (2).

Based on a survey of directors of Canadian applied health, economic, and social research organizations, the authors describe how these organizations move research into practice. The authors formulate a five-question framework for knowledge transfer within organizations. The authors suggest that research organizations should ask: "What should be transferred to decision makers?" "To whom should research knowledge be transferred?" "By whom?" "How?" and "With what effect?"

Lomas, J. 2007. "The In-Between World of Knowledge Brokering." *British Medical Journal* 334: 129–132.

Lomas serves as the CEO for the Canadian Health Services Research Foundation. The article explains the instrumental role knowledge brokers play in disseminating evidence to decision makers. The author acknowledges that neither universities nor health service providers have much motivation to maintain connections. As a result, Lomas encourages a more formal recognition of the important role that knowledge brokers play in connecting researchers and decision makers. Lomas exemplifies the role of a knowledge brokering agency by describing the activities of the CHSRF, which have helped foster an evidence-based culture. Additional resources for further research are also provided.

Shortell, S. M. 2006. "Promoting Evidence-based Management." *Frontiers of Health Services Management* **22 (3): 23–29.**

Shortell discusses the influential role of the knowledge broker in getting the right evidence for use in decisions. Knowledge brokers bridge the gap between the research community and the healthcare decision maker. Shortell sees initiatives from both the federal government and the private sector as key to furthering the field of management research. The CHSRF sponsored a knowledge-brokering evaluation in 2005. The findings can be reviewed at www.chsrf.ca/brokering/evaluation_program_e.php.

Examples of Evidence-Based Management Research

Canadian Health Services Research Foundation. 2007. "Promising Practices in Research Use." [Online information; retrieved 2/7/07.] www.chsrf.ca/promising/index_e.php.

This section of the CHSRF website recognizes institutions that have made a commitment to using evidence in their decisions. The Web page divides the cases into three categories: people, processes, and structures. The stories convey the experiences of the organizations as they tackle an issue and develop a strategy for improvement. Each case writer imparts a few pieces of advice and wisdom to the reader.

Web-Based Resources

Research Websites

General Literature Search Engines

★ Emerald Insight (www.emeraldinsight.com/Insight)
Searches 130 management journals providing full-text articles dating back to 1994

Google Scholar (scholar.google.com)
Searches of a variety of scholarly literature from a multitude of disciplines and sources

Best Practice Sources

Academy Health (www.academyhealth.org)
Health services research that collaborates with researchers, policymakers, and practitioners

Advisory Board Company (www.advisoryboardcompany.com)
Healthcare best practices research and analysis created in an environment of shared learning among about 250 leading health institutions

★ **Agency for Healthcare Research and Quality (www.ahrq. gov/research)**
Research aimed at improving outcomes, quality, cost, use, and accessibility of healthcare

Canadian Health Services Research Foundation (www.chsrf.ca)
Research on health and evidence-based management best practices. *Brokering Digest* provides clear summaries of leading evidence-based research (www.chsrf.ca/brokering/brokering_digest_e.php)

Cochrane Group (www.cochrane.org/index.htm)
Systematic reviews of outcomes of healthcare interventions

Cochrane Collaboration Effective Practice and Organization of Care Group (www.epoc.uottawa.ca)

Health Research and Educational Trust (HRET) (www.hret. org/hret_app/index.jsp)
A subsidiary of the American Hospital Association focuses on issues affecting healthcare delivery

Institute for Healthcare Improvement (www.ihi.org)
Focus on improving patient care worldwide with an emphasis on equity and efficiency

★ **Kaiser Family Foundation (www.kff.org)**
Research on the most prominent healthcare issues like Medicare/Medicaid, minority health, or the uninsured

National Institute for Health Research Service Delivery and Organization (www.sdo.lshtm.ac.uk/index.html)
Research focused on bettering the organization and delivery of health services

★ **National Library for Health (www.library.nhs.uk) Health Management Specialist site (www.library.nhs.uk/healthmanagement)**
Information specifically for health managers with news, briefings, and hot topics

National Library of Medicine Gateway (gateway.nlm.nih. gov/
gw/Cmd)
Searches of the U.S. National Library of Medicine through multiple
retrieval systems

Management Information Sources

Center for Health Management Research (www.hret.org/
hret/programs/chmr/index.html)
Provides relevant, actionable research guided by 17 member universities
and 15 industry sponsors, previously part of the University of
Washington

Evidence-Based Management (www.evidence-basedmanagement.com)
General EB management website established by professors J. Pfeffer and
R. Sutton at Stanford University

Funding Possibilities

Government Sources

Agency for Healthcare Research and Quality (www.ahrq.gov/fund/
grantix.htm)

Centers for Disease Control and Prevention Funding Opportunities
(www.cdc.gov/funding.htm)

Health Resources and Services Administration Maternal and Child
Health Bureau (www.mchb.hrsa.gov/grants)

National Institutes of Health (NIH) Bioethics Resources on the
Web (www.nih.gov/sigs/bioethics /withinnih.html#funding)

NIH National Institute on Aging (www.nia.nih.gov/funding)

NIH National Institute of Child Health and Human Development
(www.nichd.nih.gov/funding/funding.htm)

NIH National Institute of Mental Health (www.nimh.nih.gov/
grants)

NIH Office of Extramural Research Grants Home Page (grants.nih.
gov/grants/oer.htm)

National Science Foundation (www.nsf.gov/home/menus/funding.htm)

University of California Special Research Programs (www.ucop.edu/srphome)

U.S. Department of Health and Human Services Health GrantsNet (www.dhhs.gov/grantsnet/grantinfo.htm)

U.S. Department of Health and Human Services Health Resources and Services Administration (www.hrsa.gov/grants)

Private Sources

Bill and Melinda Gates Foundation
www.gatesfoundation.org

California HealthCare Foundation
www.chcf.org

Commonwealth Fund
www.cmwf.org

The Foundation Center
www.fdncenter.org

Global Forum for Health Research
www.globalforumhealth.org

The Global Fund to Fights AIDS, Tuberculosis, and Malaria
www.theglobalfund.org/en

The John A. Hartford Foundation
www.jhartfound.org

The John D. and Catherine T. MacArthur Foundation
www.macfound.org

The Pew Charitable Trusts
www.pewtrusts.com

Robert Wood Johnson Foundation
www.rwjf.org

The Rockefeller Foundation
www.rockfound.org

Soros Foundations Network and Open Society Institute
www.soros.org

W. K. Kellogg Foundation
www.wkkf.org

INDEX

Academic medical centers, evidence-based healthcare management utilization at, 17-27

AcademyHealth, website of, 86

Accelerating Change and Transformation in Organizations and Networks (ACTION) program, 14, 54, 260

Accessibility: of healthcare, 260; of research evidence, 10, 11, 13, 14, 91

Accountability: of CEOs, 154, 155; external demands for, 67-68, 70, 260; of healthcare managers, 23, 26; of hospital board members, 105; as impetus for evidence-based healthcare management, 260; for knowledge transfer, 68, 71; for pain management quality improvement, 163, 168; performance evaluations and, 112

Accuracy, of research evidence, 11, 14, 90: assessment guidelines for, 91-93; in formation of corporate universities, 143, 145, 146

ACHE (American College of Healthcare Executives), 100, 129

Acme Medical Center, inpatient bed planning at, 189-206

Acquisition, of research evidence, xxiii, 61-62, 79: for community health studies, 237-38; for depression management, 182-84; for hospital evacuation planning, 223-24; for inpatient bed planning, 190-91; for leadership development, 126-30; for pain management programs, 165-66

Actionability, of research evidence, xxiii, 10, 11, 14, 90: assessment

guidelines for, 93-94; checklist for, 242; in community health studies, 241-43; in formation of corporate universities, 143, 145, 146-47

ACTION (Accelerating Change and Transformation in Organizations and Networks) program, 14, 54, 260

Adequacy, of research evidence: assessment guidelines for, 94; checklist for, 242-43; in formation of corporate universities, 143, 145, 147

Advertisements, as source of research evidence, 87

Advisory Board Company, 37, 100, 260

Advocates, as source of research evidence, 87

Agency for Healthcare Research and Quality (AHRQ), 59, 66: Accelerating Change and Transformation in Organizations and Networks (ACTION) program, 14, 54, 260; as evidence-based healthcare management center monitor, 14; Integrated Delivery System Research Network (IDSRN), 54; as research evidence source, 61, 86, 87; research focus of, 260; website of, 86

AHRQ. *See* Agency for Healthcare Research and Quality (AHRQ)

Air transport, of patients, 228

Albert Einstein College of Medicine, 48

Alternatives, in managerial decision-making process, 60, 80

ABOUT THE AUTHORS

Anthony R. Kovner is professor of public and health management at the Wagner School of Public Service at New York University and director of the Master of Science in Management concentration for nurse leaders. An organizational theorist by training, his research interests include nurse leadership, evidence-based management, and nonprofit governance. He has been a senior manager in two hospitals, a nursing home, a group practice, and a neighborhood health center, as well as a senior healthcare consultant for a large industrial union. Professor Kovner has written 11 books and 91 peer-reviewed articles, book chapters, and case studies. His other books include *Health Services Management*, with Duncan Neuhauser (Health Administration Press, 2004); *Health Care Management in Mind: Eight Careers* (Springer, 2000); and *Health Care Delivery in the United States*, 9th edition, coeditor with James Knickman (Springer, 2008). In addition, he has been a consultant to the New York-Presbyterian Hospital, the Robert Wood Johnson Foundation, the W. K. Kellogg Foundation, Montefiore Medical Center, and the American Academy of Orthopedic Surgeons. He is a board member of the Lutheran Medical Center; is a fellow of the New York Academy of Medicine; and was director for more than 20 years of Wagner's/NYU program in health policy and management. Professor Kovner received his PhD in public administration from the University of Pittsburgh.

David J. Fine, FACHE, is president and chief executive officer of St. Luke's Episcopal Health System in Houston, Texas. Fine has 35 years of experience as a healthcare executive, including more than 25 years as chief executive officer of university hospitals, multihospital systems, medical groups, and managed care organizations. He earned a bachelor of arts degree magna cum laude from Tufts University and a Master of Hospital Administration degree from the University of Minnesota School of Public Health, where he was a U.S. Public Health Service trainee and winner of the James A. Hamilton Prize. Concurrent with his management responsibilities, Fine has held university teaching appointments for most of his career, including five years as tenured professor of health services administration and senior scholar in the Center for Outcomes and Effectiveness Research at the University of Alabama, Birmingham, and nine years as regents professor and chair of the Department of Health Systems Management at Tulane University. He is the recipient of numerous awards and honors, including a Doctor of Philosophy *Honoris Causa* from the University of Southern Mississippi in

2007. Fine is past chairman of the board of directors of the Association of University Programs in Health Administration and was founding vice-chairman of the National Center for Healthcare Leadership. He is presently a regent of the American College of Healthcare Executives.

Richard D'Aquila, FACHE, is the executive vice president and chief operating officer at Yale-New Haven Hospital and executive vice president of Yale New Haven Health System in New Haven, Connecticut. From 2000 to 2006, D'Aquila served as senior vice president and chief operating officer of New York Presbyterian Hospital/Weill Cornell Medical Center. D'Aquila also served in executive positions at St. Vincent's Medical Center in Bridgeport, Connecticut, the Mount Sinai Hospital in Hartford, Connecticut, and Health Initiatives Corporation in Providence, Rhode Island. D'Aquila received his graduate degree in hospital administration from the Yale University School of Medicine and his bachelor's degree in economics from Central Connecticut State University. He is a member of the lecturing faculty at the Wagner School of Public Service at New York University and the Yale University School of Epidemiology and Public Health.

ABOUT THE CONTRIBUTORS

Emily A. Allinder, MHA, BSBA, business manager, Saint Luke's Surgical Institute, Saint Luke's Hospital, Kansas City, MO

Laura Arroyo, research associate, Kaiser Permanente Division of Research, Oakland, CA

Patricia Gail Bray, executive director, St. Luke's Episcopal Health Charities, Houston, TX

L. Edward Bryant, attorney, Drinker Biddle & Reath, LLP, Chicago, IL

J. Brian Cassel, PhD, senior analyst, Oncology Administration, Virginia Commonwealth University Medical Center, Richmond, VA

Timothy J. Cotter, MLIR, managing director, Sullivan, Cotter and Associates, Inc., Detroit, MI

Pam Curtis, assistant director, Center for Evidence-Based Policy, Oregon Health and Science University, Portland, OR

Philip DiSalvio, BA, MEd, EdD, assistant provost, director, SetonWorldWide, Seton Hall University, South Orange, NJ

Ellen Flaherty, PhD, RN, vice president of quality improvement, Village Care of New York, New York, NY

Emily L. Garrison, BS, MHA, analyst, St. Luke's Episcopal Health System, Houston, TX

Mark Gibson, director, Center for Evidence-Based Policy, Oregon Health and Science University, Portland, OR

Ilana Graetz, PhD candidate, University of California-Berkeley, School of Public Health, Berkeley, CA

Kyle L. Grazier, PhD, editor, *Journal of Healthcare Management*, and professor, University of Michigan, Ann Arbor, MI

John Hsu, MD, MBA, MSCE, senior physician scientist, Kaiser Permanente, Oakland, CA

Peter Martelli, PhD candidate, University of California-Berkeley, School of Public Health, Berkeley, CA

Ann Scheck McAlearney, ScD, MS, associate professor, Health Services Management and Policy, College of Public Health, The Ohio State University, Columbus, OH

Rodney K. McCurdy, MHA, FACHE, doctoral candidate, Health Services and Policy Analysis program, University of California-Berkeley

K. Joanne McGlown, RN, MHHA, FACHE, PhD, president and CEO, McGlown-Self Consulting, LLC in Montevallo, AL

Sara Mody, MPA, research assistant, New York University Robert F. Wagner School of Public Service, New York, NY

William M. Murray, FACHE, president, Sisters of Charity of Leavenworth Health System, Lenexa, KS

Esther B. Neuwirth, PhD, senior manager, Center for Evaluation & Innovation, Care Management Institute, Kaiser Permanente, Oakland, CA

Stephen J. O'Connor, FACHE, director and professor, Master's of Science in Health Administration Program, Department of Health Services Administration, University of Alabama at Birmingham

Lawrence Prybil, PhD, FACHE, professor, College of Public Health, The University of Iowa, Iowa City, IA

Thomas G. Rundall, PhD, professor of health policy and management, University of California-Berkeley

Julie Schmittdiel, PhD, research scientist, Kaiser Permanente Northern California Division of Research, Oakland, CA

Richard M. Shewchuk, PhD, professor, School of Public Health, University of Alabama at Birmingham

Jancy Strauman, MN, MPH, MBA, principal, Helicon Consulting, Inc., Durham, NC

Arthur Webb, president and CEO, Village Care of New York, New York, NY

Jeffrey Weiss, MD, assistant professor of medicine and medical director, Montefiore Medical Center, Albert Einstein College of Medicine, Bronx, NY

Kenneth R. White, PhD, FACHE, Charles P. Cardwell, Jr., Professor of Health Administration, Virginia Commonwealth University, Richmond, VA

Megin Wolfman, Department of Performance Management, Yale-New Haven Hospital, New Haven, CT